DIAGNOSIS OF COLORECTAL AND OVARIAN CARCINOMA

Compliments of

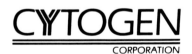

TARGETED DIAGNOSIS AND THERAPY

Editor

John D. Rodwell
Vice President, Research and Development
CYTOGEN Corporation
Princeton, New Jersey

1. Antibody-Mediated Delivery Systems, *edited by John D. Rodwell*
2. Covalently Modified Antigens and Antibodies in Diagnosis and Therapy, *edited by Gerard A. Quash and John D. Rodwell*
3. Targeted Therapeutic Systems, *edited by Praveen Tyle and Bhanu P. Ram*
4. Liver Diseases: Targeted Diagnosis and Therapy Using Specific Receptors and Ligands, *edited by George Y. Wu and Catherine H. Wu*
5. Lipoproteins as Carriers of Pharmacological Agents, *edited by Michael Shaw*
6. Diagnosis of Colorectal and Ovarian Carcinoma: Application of Immunoscintigraphic Technology, *edited by Robert T. Maguire and Douglas Van Nostrand*

ADDITIONAL VOLUMES IN PREPARATION

DIAGNOSIS OF COLORECTAL AND OVARIAN CARCINOMA

APPLICATION OF IMMUNOSCINTIGRAPHIC TECHNOLOGY

EDITED BY

ROBERT T. MAGUIRE

CYTOGEN Corporation
Princeton, New Jersey

DOUGLAS VAN NOSTRAND

Good Samaritan Hospital
Baltimore, Maryland
Uniformed Services University of Health Sciences
Bethesda, Maryland

Marcel Dekker, Inc.   New York • Basel • Hong Kong

Library of Congress Cataloging-in-Publication Data

Diagnosis of Colorectal and Ovarian Carcinoma: Application of Immuno-
scintigraphic Technology / edited by Robert T. Maguire, Douglas Van
Nostrand.
    p.   cm. -- (Targeted diagnosis and therapy; 6)
    Includes bibliographical references and index.
    ISBN 0-8247-8646-7
    1. Cancer--Radioimmunoimaging. 2. Monoclonal antibodies-
-Diagnostic use. I. Maguire, Robert T. II. Van Nostrand,
Douglas. III. Series.
    RC270.3.R33D53   1992
    616.99'40757--dc20   91-46063
                                             CIP
                                             r92

This book is printed on acid-free paper.

MARCEL DEKKER, INC.
270 Madison Avenue, New York, New York, 10016

Current printing (last digit):
10 9 8 7 6 5 4 3 2 1

PRINTED IN THE UNITED STATES OF AMERICA

Introduction to the Series

Targeted Diagnosis and Therapy is a series intended to collect new knowledge generated in the research and development of self-directed diagnostic and therapeutic agents. The powerful tools of recombinant DNA and monoclonal antibody technologies have contributed immensely to our understanding of the concept of molecular recognition as well as protein structure–function relationships. This has yielded a view of the future that includes the use of a variety of new pharmaceutical products. These products will have the property of localizing to a predetermined site, with a consequent diagnostic or therapeutic effect. The clinical use of these products will include the treatment in vivo of malignant organs or tissues as well as elimination of specific cell types in ex vivo bone marrow-purging procedures. Each volume will focus on one product or strategy, and contain the relevant preclinical and/or clinical experience. The list of near-term subjects includes a variety of antibody conjugates, the interferons, the interleukins, tissue plasminogen activator, and gene therapy. Other volumes will deal with the next generation of agents, such as genetically engineered toxins and fusion proteins. It is expected that the series will be useful for basic researchers and clinicians alike.

New frontiers lie ahead. The opportunities for research and development of important new pharmaceutical products are considerable. It is hoped that Targeted Diagnosis and Therapy will assist in the efforts to achieve this goal.

John D. Rodwell
Editor

Preface

The discovery that a variety of tumor-associated antigens are disproportionately expressed on malignant cells has led to a multitude of diagnostic and therapeutic studies using radiolabeled antibodies. Data from several large clinical trials have documented the utility of radiolabeled antibodies for presurgical staging of patients with a variety of cancers. One widely studied agent is the B72.3 murine monoclonal antibody that recognizes an antigen frequently expressed by commonly occurring adenocarcinomas. It is the goal of this volume to provide a broad overview of preclinical and clinical experience with B72.3 as a tumor-targeting agent while emphasizing results of recent studies utilizing site-specific radiolabeled B72.3 (CYT-103-[111]In: OncoScint CR103). Combining the experience of 23 authors who are experts in such diverse fields as immunology, pharmacology, medical and surgical oncology, and radiology and nuclear medicine, this book provides insight into the generation and subsequent development of monoclonal antibodies as clinically useful reagents.

In the first chapter, Halpern gives an overview of monoclonal antibody technology and radioimmunodetection methodology. He points out progress made to date but stresses the many areas for further research in the field. In Chapter 2, Colcher et al. describe the generation of the B72.3 monoclonal antibody and review the extensive preclinical evaluation of this reagent, while in the third chapter, Carrasquillo describes the original clinical experience with radioiodinated B72.3 — trials that laid the groundwork for future development of OncoScint CR103. Lastoria and Salvatore (Chapter 4) describe the European clinical experience with radiolabeled B72.3 and provide insight into the potential clinical utility of immunoscintigraphy.

Chapters 5 and 6 deal with the multicenter clinical trial results with ^{111}In-labeled B72.3 (OncoScint CR103) and the documented impact on patient management of immunoscintigraphic studies with this product. Chapters 7 and 8 review the OncoScint clinical trial results in patients with ovarian cancer and demonstrate the strong impact of antibody imaging on the care of patients with this tumor type. Chapters 5 through 8 also emphasize specific patient subgroups in which immunoscintigraphy is most useful. It is pointed out that immunoscintigraphy is often complementary to standard diagnostic procedures used for the diagnosis and staging of cancer. Antibody imaging provides whole-body information that can be useful in directing subsequent diagnostic procedures.

A detailed OncoScint image atlas is given in Chapter 9. Examples of normal radiolabeled antibody biodistribution, primary and recurrent colorectal and ovarian tumor localization, and potential pitfalls in image interpretation are included. In Chapter 10, reviews of the pharmacokinetics of indium-labeled B72.3 provide a physiological basis for the patterns of distribution noted in the previous chapter. Chapter 11 provides a very useful description of the practical aspects of image acquisition with OncoScint. This chapter presents detailed information on radiolabeling, gamma camera quality control, and image acquisition parameters (including SPECT parameters) necessary for optimal use of the product. In the final chapter, McKearn provides an overview of likely future developments in the field of radioimmunodetection.

It is hoped that this comprehensive review of immunoscintigraphy, and OncoScint in particular, will be of use to clinicians caring for patients with cancer in addition to investigators interested in pursuing this area of research.

The editors are grateful to the contributors for their efforts in reviewing of their individual subject areas. We would also like to express our sincere appreciation to the staff at Marcel Dekker, Inc., who assisted with a high degree of professionalism. Finally, we deeply appreciate the contributions of Dr. Virginia Pascucci and Ms. Dolores Dunsker, without whose efforts this book would not have been completed.

Robert T. Maguire
Douglas Van Nostrand

Contents

Series Introduction   *iii*

Preface   *v*

Contributors   *ix*

1. An Overview of Radioimmunoimaging   1
    Samuel E. Halpern

2. Generation and Characterization of Monoclonal Antibody B72.3:
    Experimental and Preclinical Studies   23
    David M. Colcher, Diane E. Milenic, and Jeffrey Schlom

3. Imaging of Colorectal Carcinoma with ^{131}I B72.3 Monoclonal Antibody   45
    Jorge A. Carrasquillo

4. Monoclonal Antibody B72.3 Immunoscintigraphy in the Follow-Up of
    Patients with Colorectal Cancer   57
    Secondo Lastoria and Marco Salvatore

5. Multicenter Clinical Trials of Monoclonal Antibody B72.3-GYK-DPTA-
    ^{111}In (^{111}In-CYT-103; OncoScint CR103) in Patients with Colorectal
    Carcinoma   73
    Hani H. Abdel-Nabi and Ralph J. Doerr

6. OncoScint CR103 Imaging in the Surgical Management of Patients
    with Colorectal Cancer   89
    Ralph J. Doerr and Hani H. Abdel-Nabi

7. Multicenter Clinical Trial of ^{111}In-CYT-103 in Patients with
    Ovarian Cancer   111
    Donald G. Gallup

8. Impact of ^{111}In-CYT-103 on the Surgical Management of Patients
    with Ovarian Cancer   125
    Earl A. Surwit

9. OncoScint Image Atlas   141
    Robert T. Maguire

10. Immunopharmacokinetics of ^{111}In-CYT-103 in Ovarian Cancer Patients   177
    William J. Jusko, Li-Pin Kung, and Raymond F. Schmelter

11. A Practical Approach to Planar and SPECT Imaging of ^{111}In-CYT-103   191
    *B. David Collier, LisaAnn Trembath, Yu Liu, H. Turgut Turoglu,
    Neetin Patel and Shekhar Thakur*

12. Future Directions in Tumor Radioimmunodetection   211
    Thomas J. McKearn

Index   223

Contributors

Hani H. Abdel-Nabi, M.D., Ph.D. *Associate Professor, Department of Nuclear Medicine, State University of New York at Buffalo, Buffalo, New York*

Jorge A. Carrasquillo, M.D. *Deputy Chief, Department of Nuclear Medicine, Clinical Center, National Cancer Institute, National Institutes of Health, Bethesda, Maryland*

David M. Colcher, Ph.D.* *Laboratory of Tumor Immunology and Biology, National Cancer Institute, National Institutes of Health, Bethesda, Maryland*

B. David Collier, M.D. *Professor, Department of Radiology, and Director, Section of Nuclear Medicine, Medical College of Wisconsin, Milwaukee, Wisconsin*

Ralph J. Doerr, M.D. Associate Professor, Department of Surgery, and Assistant Professor, Department of Nuclear Medicine, State University of New York at Buffalo, Buffalo, New York

---

*Present Affiliation: *Professor, Department of Pathology and Microbiology, University of Nebraska Medical Center, Omaha, Nebraska*

Donald G. Gallup, M.D. *Professor, Section of Gynecological Oncology, Department of Obstetrics and Gynecology, Medical College of Georgia, Augusta, Georgia*

Samuel E. Halpern, M.D. *Chief, Nuclear Medicine Service, Department of Nuclear Medicine, Veterans Administration Medical Center, and Professor, Department of Radiology, University of California at San Diego, San Diego, California*

William J. Jusko, Ph.D. *Professor, Department of Pharmaceutics, State University of New York at Buffalo, Buffalo, New York*

Li-Pin Kung, B.S. *Research Assistant, Department of Pharmaceutics, State University of New York at Buffalo, Buffalo, New York*

Secondo Lastoria, M.D. *Professor, Department of Nuclear Medicine, University of Naples, 2nd Medical School, and Department of Nuclear Medicine, National Cancer Institute, "G. Pascale," Naples, Italy*

Yu Liu, M.D. *Resident Physician, Department of Nuclear Medicine, Medical College of Wisconsin, Milwaukee, Wisconsin*

Robert T. Maguire, M.D. *Director, Department of Clinical Investigations, CYTOGEN Corporation, Princeton, New Jersey*

Thomas J. McKearn, M.D., Ph.D. *President, CYTOGEN Corporation, Princeton, New Jersey*

Diane E. Milenic, M.S. *Laboratory of Tumor Immunology and Biology, National Cancer Institute, National Institutes of Health, Bethesda, Maryland*

Neetin Patel, M.D. *Resident Physician, Department of Nuclear Medicine, Medical College of Wisconsin, Milwaukee, Wisconsin*

Marco Salvatore, M.D. *Professor, Department of Nuclear Medicine, University of Naples, 2nd Medical School, and Scientific Director, Department of Nuclear Medicine, National Cancer Institute, "G. Pascale," Naples, Italy*

Jeffrey Schlom, Ph.D. *Chief, Laboratory of Tumor Immunology and Biology, National Cancer Institute, National Institutes of Health, Bethesda, Maryland*

Raymond F. Schmelter, Ph.D. *Associate Director, Department of Pharmaceutical Development, CYTOGEN Corporation, Princeton, New Jersey*

Earl A. Surwit, M.D. *Professor, Department of Obstetrics/Gynecology and Surgery, University of Arizona, Tucson, Arizona*

Shekhar Thakur, M.D. *Resident Physician, Department of Nuclear Medicine, Medical College of Wisconsin, Milwaukee, Wisconsin*

LisaAnn Trembath, B.S., C.N.M.T. *Nuclear Medicine Research Technologist, and Research Coordinator, Medical College of Wisconsin, Milwaukee, Wisconsin*

H. Turgut Turoglu, M.D. *Research Assistant, Department of Nuclear Medicine, Faculty of Medicine, Marmara University, Istanbul, Turkey*

1

An Overview of Radioimmunoimaging

Samuel E. Halpern
Veterans Affairs Medical Center, San Diego, California

INTRODUCTION

Radioimmunoimaging is no longer a new area of investigation even though, at the time of this writing, the field is still awaiting its first American commercial radioimmunodetection (RID) product. The pioneers began work nearly 40 years ago, when Pressman and co-workers immunized a mouse against a murine tumor, isolated the antibody, iodinated it, injected it into a mouse bearing a murine tumor that carried the antigen, and demonstrated antigen targeting at levels beyond those which could be accounted for on a nonspecific basis [1,2]. Between 1950 and 1990, investigators in this field encountered many obstacles in bringing RID into clinical reality.

Until recently, little was known about antibodies or their antigen targets. In the majority of cases, the molecular weight of the antigen was unknown, as well as its location in or on the tumor cell. Nothing was known about the rate of antigen production or whether it varied from antigen to antigen or remained in stable production within the same tumor. The mechanisms that turned antigen production on or off were a mystery, as was the antigenic secretory rate of the tumor. Moreover, the distribution of the antigen in the normal tissues of the human body was generally unknown, although it was realized that normal tissues could produce such antigens. For example, carcinoembryonic antigen (CEA), the most thoroughly researched of the tumor-associated antigens, is produced by the normal colon. This raises the question of the potential consequences of normal tissue antigen expression on the distribution of an exogenously administered radiolabeled antibody.

In the early years, the distribution of antigen on tumor cells also was largely unknown. Subsequent research indicated that antigen distribution varied markedly from tumor system to tumor system and even within an individual metastasis. The steric configuration of antigens was also unknown. Furthermore, no one knew what would happen to the immune complex as a result of an antigen:antibody interaction at the tissue level. Most of the issues noted here regarding the target antigen remain inadequately explored today.

As with antigens, little was known about antibodies. Until the 1970s, no one was really sure what would happen if multimilligram quantities of a murine IgG were infused into a human. In fact, since in vivo immune complex formation was known to cause life-threatening disease, the administration of mouse protein into human subjects was believed to constitute a considerable risk. The distribution of a radiolabeled murine antibody in a human subject was, of course, totally unknown.

Potential toxicity and antibody distribution were not the only issues. The importance of the affinity of an antibody for effective RID was and continues to be a mystery. The importance and even the reality of avidity is still in question, and, as yet, there is no generally accepted definition for this term.

The configuration of the antibody, its class, subclass, and the effect of the quantity and position of the carbohydrate groups on its in vivo distribution all remained to be determined. Further, investigators knew (and know) very little about how the antigen and the antibody interact at the level of the tumor or what the stability of such a complex would be in view of the aberrant physiology of the tumor. In fact, the whole question of the physiology and pharmacology of high-molecular-weight proteins at the tumor and normal tissue level is not well researched from the standpoint of our technology.

Finally, there is the question of which isotope is best suited for the purpose of RID. This has not been solved to the satisfaction of many researchers.

As described, numerous questions and potential problems are associated with RID; however, a great deal of progress has been made in this field during the past 40 years. The history of RID as well as the current status of this area are reviewed herein.

THE BEGINNING
Origin of the Immune System

It is generally accepted that the immune system began developing about 300,000,000 years ago [3]. The first animals exhibiting the rudimentary system were probably the immediate ancestors of the vertebrates [3]. For animals lower than the vertebrates in the phylogenetic order, it is difficult to completely define an immune system. The mammals, of course, all have an extraordinary immune system. In the mammals, there are five classes of antibodies, varying in size from the smallest (IgG), weighing about 150,000 daltons, to the giant IgM, with an estimated weight of over 900,000 daltons [4]. There is a species difference in antibodies, of course, yet their similarities are more obvious than their differences. The cells that manufacture the antibodies in various species are similar; these cells go through similar juvenile, adult, and aging stages; and they can even degenerate into the same malignancies. The polyclonal antibodies used in RID have been raised in many species. Goats, sheep, horses, and pigs have all supplied their antibody mixtures for research purposes. This has not been the case with monoclonal antibodies, as we shall see. Most of the imaging that has been done has utilized the IgG variety of antibody; however, IgMs have sometimes been utilized [5,6].

The IgG Molecule

The IgG molecule is schematically represented by the letter "Y." In reality, it looks more like a coiled spring. An even more accurate description would be obtained from twisting and wrapping the spring in on itself in the general shape of a Y. This Y configuration is really observed only when the antibody interacts with the antigen. In its noninteractive state, IgGs appear somewhat globular. An IgG is constructed of modules composed of two light chains and two heavy chains linked together by disulfide bridges. A total of about 1200 amino acids are involved [3,4]. The molecule can be dissected by enzymatic digestion to produce component parts. The stem of the Y (also known as the Fc) can be produced by papain treatment. The Fc weighs about 50,000 daltons and is made from two identical parts of the heavy chain. It is unique in that it carries nearly all the carbohydrate for the entire molecule, although occasionally an IgG will have a small sugar component above this level. The Fc is more or less constant in structure, as opposed to the rest of the antibody [3,4]. In fact, it is so constant it can be crystallized and receives its name, F-C (Fragment Crystalline) due to this phenomenon.

The specific immunoreactive areas of the IgG reside on the fragment antigen binding (Fab) portion of the molecule. The Fab weighs approximately 50,000 daltons and represents one-third of the antibody molecule. Part of the Fab is relatively unchanged from antibody to antibody, while a second section, the "variable" region, varies among different antibodies. On the variable portion, yet another region, known as the hypervariable region, is characterized by considerable variability. There are three hypervariable regions on the variable portion of the Fab. Altogether the variable regions make up 25% of the amino acids of a Fab and, as such, allow an incredible number of interactive permutations. Two such Fab areas bridged together are known as a F(ab')2 (100,000 daltons) and account for up to two-thirds of the total mass of the antibody protein and convey its overall specificity.

Any theory of RID that does not take into account the vast size and complexity of the IgG molecule is doomed to failure. These molecules are not only large steric entities, but they also carry a charge [4]. This charge may vary from monoclonal antibody to monoclonal antibody. Some IgGs have a low isoelectric point, while others fall well above 7.0. This uniqueness, of course, is brought about by the charged amino acids in the body of the molecule. Living cells (parts of them anyway) also carry a charge. The capillaries of the kidney, for example, carry a negative charge [7]. Consider what might happen if a positively charged molecule of 50,000 daltons traversed them [7,8]. The molecule could be attracted to the surface of the capillary endothelium with possible enhancement of its renal clearance [9].

Overall, antibodies are huge, complex proteins and, therefore, present numerous difficulties for RID researchers who attempt to attach complex molecules to the antibody structure for clinical purposes.

Production of a Monoclonal Antibody

The manufacture of an antibody by nature is a complex process. First, the assembly plant itself (the B lymphocyte) and its eventual progeny (the plasma cell) must be built. This is a complicated process involving cell production and maturation. In adults, the B lymphocyte is produced in the bone marrow in great numbers. When these cells leave the marrow, they travel to the lymph nodes or spleen. The cells then face a life crisis. If they are stimulated by an antigen, they can transform into plasma cells and begin to secrete antibody, or they can choose to divide and become "memory B cells." These cells have the special characteristic of producing a rapid response if the same antigen challenges the organism a second time. If the lymphocyte is never stimulated by an antigen, it remains a "virgin" cell [4] and dies quickly. However, the plasma cell is also short-lived. It lasts only a matter of weeks, but during this time it is a heavy producer of antibodies. The B cell can also produce antibody. A single B lymphocyte will produce only a single type of antibody. Thus, if the B cell could be harvested, cloned, and immortalized, it would produce a monoclonal antibody. Through the genius of Kohler and Milstein we now have the means to produce such entities [12].

As can be deduced from the above discussion, when invaders enter the body they are "seen" by a large number of B lymphocytes. These cells are activated, each manufacturing its unique product. The end result of this is a variety of antibodies, which differ in affinity, charge, avidity, and probably distribution if injected into a human subject. These antibodies do not have "predefined specificity" [12]. This lack of specificity is fine as far as the body's defenses are concerned, but for the purposes of RID, a highly selective antibody with a particular affinity, charge, stability, and so forth — in short, a monoclonal antibody — is required [12].

Monoclonal antibodies are produced by the creation of hybrid cells called hybridomas. The production process is highly complicated. For a detailed description of the technology, the reader is referred to an excellent chapter on the subject by Kearney et al. [13]. While the efforts of Kohler and Milstein [12] were critical in this work, experiments by Potter and others [14–18] were important to their success. The work by Potter [14,15] produced transplantable mouse myelomas in abundance. A tremendous amount was learned about the function of such cells from these unique cancers. Cell fusion technology [16–18] was just as critical, because without the ability to fuse cells, hybridomas could not exist.

Kohler and Milstein [12], of course, knew of this earlier work and used myeloma cells and fusion technology to form the hybridomas. In the manufacture of a hybridoma for antibody production, it is important to carefully select both the malignant immortalizing cell and the specific B lymphocyte to be used for the fusion. The selection of the correct myeloma cell is important because many of these cells are known to produce both heavy and light chains. Fusion with such a cell could result in hybrid antibodies. Such a hybrid would obviously have a diminished ability to bind to the antigen. Ideally, light and heavy chains would be produced exclusively from the B lymphocyte gene code. For this reason, one selects a myeloma cell that has lost the ability to make its own light and heavy chains. The actual selection process is subtle and beyond the scope of this chapter.

The production of the sensitized B lymphocyte results from immunization of the murine host with the antigen. The mouse is generally injected multiple times with the antigen. Next, the animal's spleen is removed and its cells prepared for fusion with the "nonsecreting" immortal myeloma cell. Multiple immunization procedures have been used in this process, since the route of inoculation can alter the production characteristics of the B lymphocytes.

After the myeloma cells and the B lymphocytes have been harvested, they are placed together in approximately equal numbers in a tube and centrifuged at 37°C. Then the cells are incubated in a solution of polyethylene glycol and again centrifuged. A variety of compounds are often added to enhance the effectiveness of this process. The end result of this attempted fusion is plated out onto culture plates. Only about 1 in 10,000 possible fusions actually take place and become apparent in nine or ten days. One problem with the technique is the need to kill any unfused myeloma cells. If this is not done, the myeloma cells overwhelm the whole process. This selective killing is accomplished during the hybridization by the use of "HAT" compounds. Three weeks after plating, antibody production can be observed. Once the hybridomas are functioning, the cells can be grown in the peritoneal cavity of a mouse or in tissue culture.

There are many caveats to this technology. For example, there are good and bad antibody producers. Obviously, for industrial purposes, a good producer is necessary. The type of immunoglobulin produced is another variable. Some cells will be IgG producers, while others produce IgMs. IgGs are preferred for RID work and, therefore, IgG-producing cells are used for the fusion.

HISTORY OF IMMUNOSCINTIGRAPHY

Following the work of Pressman et al., a great deal of animal work was directed toward RID [19-24]. It could be consistently shown that there was greater tumor uptake of the specific antibody as compared to nonspecific antibody. Double-label experiments [23], with one tracer on the nonspecific and a different tracer on the specific antibody, and experiments in which both specific and nonspecific tumors were utilized in the same mice were performed [24]. Generally, there was 2-4 times as much of the radionuclide in the specific tumor as in the nonspecific tumor.

In 1978, Goldenberg et al. [25] published one of the two most important early papers on RID in humans. By targeting CEA with ^{131}I-labeled polyclonal antibodies, this group was able to detect over 80% of the lesions in patients whose tumors presumably bore the antigen. Two years later, a Swiss group headed by Mach [26] published the second important paper, in which they reported results inferior to those of Goldenberg with a radioiodinated polyclonal anti-CEA product. Mach et al. could image only about 40% of the lesions. They concluded that the technique lacked the required sensitivity to be of clinical utility. Antibodies directed toward other tumors were studied with variable results. While these studies were being published, investigators were anxious to begin work with monoclonal antibodies. Mach et al. [27] reported improved results with monoclonal antibodies compared to their findings using polyclonal antibodies. However, it was difficult to ascertain whether this improvement was due to the use of monoclonal antibodies or to technical improvements in image acquisition.

During these early imaging investigations, "subtraction" techniques were frequently utilized. That is, the patient would be positioned for the scan, and after the imaging, a second radiopharmaceutical, often labeled albumin, would be injected. The theory was that if the nonspecific radiolabel marked the blood pool, areas of increased uptake outside the blood pool would have a greater chance of corresponding to a specific site of uptake. To some extent this was true. Unfortunately, subtraction techniques are difficult to perform perfectly, and unless the technology works well, they can cause confusion in scan interpretation. It was obvious even then that a diminution in background was more important than electronic manipulation of the data, although the latter is not without merit. Shortly after Mach's 1981 paper, Larson et al. began using monoclonal antitumor antibodies for clinical studies [28]. Other investigators in this field included Britton and Granowska in the United Kingdom. Britton's work utilized a radioiodinated monoclonal antibody targeting a human milk fat globulin antigen (HMFG-2) found on several cancers. This group utilized a unique type of subtraction technique, which involved imaging the patient within minutes after injection. During subsequent scans, the investigators simply observed uptake of the radiopharmaceutical and compared it with uptake observed in the earlier image [29]. This group was able to detect greater than 80% of the known tumor lesions using this approach.

Larson et al. [30], using ^{131}I-Fab fragments of a monoclonal antimelanoma antibody, were able to detect 85–90% of the known melanoma lesions in a small series of patients. They also indicated that there was a direct relationship between the amount of antigen on the tumor and the ability to detect the tumor with RID.

Mach and Delaloye et al. [31,32] began working extensively with I-123-labeled Fabs in the early 1980s and were able to detect about 90% of known colon lesions with this antibody fragment. This group considered the detection rate and image quality to be improved when a Fab fragment was used as the imaging molecule. F(ab')2 was also studied by these investigators, but they considered Fab to be their fragment of choice [32].

In many monoclonal antibody imaging studies, radioiodine has been employed as the tracer [25–32]. In general, these studies have indicated a sensitivity of at least 70%. However, even as the iodinated antibody studies were showing improved results, it became obvious to investigators that there might be better tracers for this work.

RADIONUCLIDE ALTERNATIVES TO ISOTOPES OF IODINE
What Is Wrong with Iodine?

Radioiodination is so much a part of the history of radiolabeled antibodies for RID that it is almost a tradition. Indeed, an isotope of iodine was used by Pressman in his initial studies [1,2]. The radiolabeling of other proteins prior to the work of Pressman and his co-workers was also done by iodination. Even nature iodinates organic compounds for pharmacological purposes in the formation of thyroid hormone. Not only can the thyroid gland apply the element to thyronine, but the peripheral tissues are capable of removing the same atom from the molecule. The process of iodination can be accomplished just as easily in the chemistry laboratory by enzymatic (lactoperoxidase) technique [33] or the time-tested chloramine T reaction [34]. Recently, Wilbur et al. [35] have developed additional iodination techniques for proteins that may confer a greater stability on the labeled molecule.

With so many methods available and the techniques so well known that they can be utilized by virtually any investigator, it is obvious why iodination quickly became the dominant method for radiolabeling antibodies for RID. Unfortunately, certain problems with the technique were ignored or not completely researched. It was known, for example, that overiodination of a protein would result in problems with its biological effectiveness. It was also known that administration of an iodinated compound to a human or an animal required that the thyroid gland be blocked to prevent it from accumulating iodine. This observation should have alerted researchers to possible problems with stability of radioiodinated antibodies. Moreover, if one peruses the data from the early animal and human RID studies and tries to account for all the administered activity, it becomes obvious that much of the radiolabel cannot be accounted for. This potential problem was ignored.

We repeated some of the radioiodine-labeled antibody studies in murine tumor models, and we continue to be puzzled by the results. First, some of the labeling methods, such as the Hunter-Boulton method, appear to be quite unstable [36]. With this approach, the iodine came off the antibody molecule within a day after labeling. Other methods, such as the lactoperoxidase method, seemed to result in stable products for about 24 hrs; at later times, however, there was continuous and progressive breakdown in most tissues [37,38]. Further, there seemed to be a difference in the rate of dehalogenation in various normal tissues, especially in the liver, which apparently has a very vigorous dehalogenation process. In addition, certain antibodies appear to dehalogenate faster than others. In fact, one antimelanoma antibody studied in our laboratory was found to have extraordinary stability, with virtually no dehalogenation.

Dehalogenation is not the only problem that characterizes radioiodination. The isotopes themselves leave something to be desired in the clinical setting. Only two isotopes of iodine, ^{123}I and ^{131}I, are useful for RID purposes. In the case of the ^{123}I, the 13.3-hr. half-life virtually requires all imaging to be completed within the first 36 hrs. If the studies are delayed much longer than this, the time needed to acquire diagnostic images increases considerably unless one acquires fewer counts. If the latter path is chosen, counting statistics become a major issue.

Imaging within the first 36 hrs. after administration of intact antibody product is problematic because the background has not diminished to the extent necessary to produce effective lesion-to-background ratios. Thus, ^{123}I is primarily used with antibody fragments, especially the small Fab fragment. Even when the Fab fragment is used, counting statistics become a problem because clearance of Fab from the body is much faster than clearance of the intact antibody. Less than 1 mCi of the [123]I Fab' is left in the body 24 hr after injection of 5mCi into the patient. Under these circumstances, required imaging times are long, and single photon emission tomography (SPECT), which is also highly statistics dependent, cannot be optimally performed. Nonetheless, of the isotopes of iodine, ^{123}I has the best characteristics for gamma camera imaging, having a 159 Kev photon, being monoenergetic, delivering little in the way of radiation dose to the patient, and allowing use of low-energy collimation.

I-131 has been the most commonly used radioisotope for RID for many years [39,40]. Unfortunately, it is a poor isotope for gamma camera imaging. First, the 364 Kev photon and the other higher-energy photons produced by the decay of the atom require high-energy collimation. The crystal efficiency for ^{131}I is about 20%, a value associated with a dramatic reduction in the number of photons counted. The radiation dose from ^{131}I is very significant, mostly due to the 600 Kev beta particles produced in its decay scheme. Obviously, the thyroid must be blocked, or any iodine that is removed from the antibody could be accumulated by the organ. Finally, the 8-day physical half-life is much longer than needed for RID. Since only modest amounts of ^{131}I can be administered to a patient because of high radiation doses, and given the poor crystal efficiency and need for high-energy collimation, the imaging time for ^{131}I becomes long and the resolution of the lesion poor. A combination of the above problems led chemists to develop other tracers and other methods for labeling antibodies.

Alternatives—[111]In and [99m]Tc

The only other radiopharmaceuticals utilized extensively for RID have been ^{111}In and [99m]Tc. Work with ^{111}In began in the early 1980s [36–38, 40–43]l Because direct application of ^{111}In to the antibody was not feasible, bifunctional chelation techniques were used. One of the more celebrated techniques for the labeling of proteins was introduced by Krejcarek and Tucker in the late 1970s [44]; the methodology was later advanced by Meares and his group [43]. Early methods involved use of the chelator DTPA, which is capable of efficiently binding [111]In. DTPA has five carboxyl groups. One of the carboxyls on the DTPA molecule can be converted to the anhydride, which then can be made, under the correct conditions, to react with lysine groups on the antibody molecule. If care is taken to control the proportion of antibody to anhydride in the reaction mixture, a situation can be achieved where the antibody carries only one or two DTPA side chains. The antibody plus ligand is then column-purified, placed in a buffer, and prepared for labeling with [111]In. Some commercial manufacturers produce the product in a kit form, which can be reconstituted on site. Any unattached ^{111}In can be removed by adding free DTPA to the kit, thereby sequestering all unbound [111]In. The ^{111}In-DTPA is then excreted rapidly through the kidney via glomerular filtration. The technique described is only one of several that can be used for ^{111}In labeling. Placing the side chain on the carbohydrate groups of the antibody is another popular and successful method [45]. Theoretically, this latter chelation method confers greater stability on the ^{111}In-antibody complex and may help retain immunoreactivity.

[111]In has several advantages for RID. It does not dehalogenate, and any ^{111}In that does come off the molecule is not concentrated by the thyroid gland. The two principal photons of [111]In (173 and 247 Kev) are low enough in energy that medium-energy collimation can be used for imaging. Further, the interaction of these photons with the gamma camera crystal is such that one achieves nearly one count by the gamma camera for each atom that decays. This results in a high photon flux if 5 mCi is administered. Moreover, since ^{111}In has a 2.8-day half-life, the patient can, if necessary, be studied multiple times during the course of a week. SPECT is also accomplished easily following the administration of ^{111}In-labeled antibodies.

The ^{111}In technique is not without problems, however. The liver accumulates ^{111}In either as the free radionuclide or as the radiolabeled antibody. As a consequence, up to 15–20% of the ^{111}In has been demonstrated to accumulate in this organ following administration of intact antibody [46]. This can make it difficult to image metastatic disease in this organ.

The most commonly used of all radionuclides in nuclear medicine is [99m]Tc. This has led to the attempted use of this isotope to label antibodies for RID [47–49]. Positive imaging results have been achieved clinically using ^{99m}Tc-labeled Fab [50,51]. The Fritzberg labeling method produces a compound that is cleared rapidly from the vascular compartment and enters the tumor quickly, especially in the form of a Fab fragment. Very little of the radionuclide is seen in the liver. The preponderance of the ^{99m}Tc-Fab is found in the kidneys, making it somewhat difficult to detect tumor contiguous with these organs. If it could be made to function well with monoclonal antibodies, ^{99m}Tc would be nearly the ideal radioisotope for RID. It can be generator-produced on site, eluted, and concentrated to an extraordinary specific activity, and it delivers very little in the way of a radiation dose per millicurie. It can be used with low-energy collimation, and its 140 Kev photon has a nearly 100% interaction with the gamma camera crystal. Its cost per millicurie is low when compared with ^{111}In or any of the isotopes of iodine. It is possible to achieve an extremely high photon flux because the radionuclide can be administered in such great quantities. The problem encountered with ^{99m}Tc involves its 6-hr. half-life. Imaging must be performed within an 18-to-24-hr. time frame. Under these circumstances, one may be limited to the use of a Fab fragment, since the F(ab')2 and the intact molecule theoretically are not cleared fast enough from the vascular compartment to allow acquisition of diagnostic images. Moreover, the high renal uptake of ^{99m}Tc-Fab makes abdominal imaging somewhat difficult. Interestingly, Baum et al [52] report excellent imaging results using a ^{99m}Tc-labeled *intact* antibody. If these data are reproducible, ^{99m}Tc could become the most important of the immune imaging radionuclides.

There is a caveat to this discussion of the radionuclides for RID that must be borne in mind. It is desirable to bring the use of antibody technology into the therapy field. As such, it would be desirable to develop a labeling technique with a gamma emitter that would predict the kinetics and distribution of the same antibody labeled with a therapeutic isotope. In the case of ^{123}I, the therapeutic counterpart would be ^{131}I, with the expectation that the pharmacology of an iodine-labeled antibody would be similar for all iodine isotopes. In the case of ^{111}In, the proposed therapeutic counterpart has been ^{90}Y, a beta emitter of great energy. Work in our laboratory indicates that the two labels can be made to perform nearly the same way in vivo when attached to the antibody, thus producing a "matched pair." This process requires sophisticated chemistry and much trial and error, however, because the two elements are not even members of the same family on the periodic table.

In the case of ^{99m}Tc, the therapeutic counterpart becomes an isotope of rhenium. Rhenium and technetium have similar chemical properties and chelation characteristics, making the chemistry somewhat easier than in the case of ^{90}Y and ^{111}In. From the gamma emitter data, it is possible to calculate the radiation dose delivered by the therapeutic ion to the tumor and normal organs.

Imaging with the Alternatives ^{111}In and ^{99m}Tc

As discussed, ^{111}In has become a popular radionuclide for RID purposes. Studies in multiple tumor systems involving a variety of antigens have been performed using ^{111}In-labeled monoclonal antibodies [6,53–56]. ^{111}In has been attached to intact antibodies as well as F(ab')2, Fab, and Fab' fragments. The sensitivity, specificity, and accuracy of these studies have varied for several reasons. The first variable has been the antibody utilized. Our group has studied breast, colon, lung, and prostate carcinoma, melanoma, medullary thyroid carcinoma, and lymphoma tumors in over 200 patients using intact antibody. Approximately 20 different antibodies have been utilized, three of which were IgM (of human origin) and the rest were murine IgGs. Tumor was targeted with all these antibodies, with some being highly successful, others unsuccessful. Our overall results in colon cancer, using intact antibody, have been in the range of 70% sensitivity for lesions 1.5 cm or greater in size. Disappointing results were observed in prostate cancer patients using antibodies that targeted the prostate-specific and prostatic acid phosphatase antigens.

Our findings using ^{111}In-labeled anti-CEA antibody have been reproduced in other laboratories [57,58]; indeed, the overall detection rates observed by other investigators may be somewhat higher than we achieved. The problem areas have included the liver, in which the accumulation of ^{111}In in the normal tissue has made it difficult to develop lesion-to-background ratios high enough to detect the tumor [57]. SPECT has been helpful in this area, but even with tomographic imaging, lesions can be missed in the liver under the best of circumstances. Moreover, SPECT imaging sometimes results in false positive readings in this organ [59].

Mass Effects

An interesting observation is the difference in the sensitivities of various antibodies and their relationship to the mass of carrier antibody administered. This so-called "carrier effect" [53,54] is highly important because it can alter not just the organ distribution of the radiopharmaceutical, but also its serum half-time. It must be remembered that uptake of the radiolabeled antibody by the tumor is limited by the amount of radiopharmaceutical delivered to the lesion. Some antibodies can be administered intravenously in very low quantities and yet exhibit long serum half-lives. Others will show a dramatic clearing from the blood and compartmentalization in the liver, spleen, bone, and other organs. When increasing quantities of unlabeled antibody are administered, the serum half-lives of these latter antibodies will often lengthen. Under such circumstances, liver metastases, which ordinarily appear as photopenic defects, can be seen as areas of increased uptake. Thus, the carrier effect is real, but variable in degree, and dependent on which antibody is administered. The etiology of this mass effect is thought to be saturation of "nonspecific" binding sites in various organs, but it is not known exactly which sites are involved and why the effect should vary from antibody to antibody.

INTACT ANTIBODY VERSUS FRAGMENTS FOR RID

We have been fortunate in our laboratory to have been able to study the same ^{111}In-labeled antibody (ZCE-025) in its intact, F(ab')2, and Fab' form [60]. ZCE-025 has an affinity of approximately 6×10^9 moles per liter and forms the F(ab')2 fragment quite well with standard digestion [61]. Imaging times for intact and F(ab')2 ZCE-025 ranged from 72 to 144 hrs., whereas imaging with the Fab' species was performed at 72 hr. In these studies, 5 mCi of ^{111}In was administered and the mass of carrier antibody ranged from 20 to 40 mg. The intact antibody had a serum half-time of approximately 48 hr., the F(ab')2 between 24 and 36 hr., and the Fab' between 12 and 24 hr. The liver showed the most intense concentration of ^{111}In following administration of intact antibody. Liver uptake was lower but kidney activity was increased when F(ab')2 was administered. The kidney becomes the target organ with ^{111}In Fab' administration, whereas liver concentration diminishes dramatically. Small lesions in the liver became positive when ^{111}In Fab' was administered. Chest lesions, especially in the mediastinum, are easier to detect with the radiolabeled fragments than with intact antibody. Overall, we detected approximately 70% of the lesions with intact antibody, over 80% with the F(ab')2, and greater than 90% with the Fab'. Many putative lesions were observed in these studies, with increased numbers being detected with the fragments than with the intact molecule. Only 10 patients were studied with the Fab', but it became obvious that lesions were observed earlier with the Fab' than with the intact molecule.

The case for ^{99m}Tc-labeled RID is predicated on its low cost per millicurie and its many favorable physical characteristics. The isotope suffers, however, from its 6-hr. physical half-life, which limits the time available for serial imaging. Yet, the data from ^{99m}Tc antibody studies indicate that when ^{99m}Tc coordination is achieved by the Fritzberg technique, worthwhile results can be obtained. This labeling technique appears to permit a very rapid clearance of ^{99m}Tc-Fab complex from the vascular compartment. This technique results in a more rapid clearance than that observed by our group using a ^{99m}Tc-labeled Fab in which the radiolabel was applied to the antibody by a different chelation technique. In our clinical studies, the kinetics and organ distribution of ^{99m}Tc Fab were virtually identical to those of the ^{111}In-labeled Fab product. That is to say, 20–25% of the injected dose remained in the vascular compartment 24 hr. after injection, resulting in problems with imaging.

The potential for ^{99m}Tc to be used in the so-called "hapten" imaging system, however, has intriguing possibilities [62]. In this scenario, the patient is administered a hybrid antibody, in which one of the variable groups is specific for a low-molecular-weight (<1000 daltons) molecule that carries the radiolabel (the hapten), while the other Fab is specific for the antigen on the tumor. Time is allowed for this antibody to be acquired by the tumor and cleared from the serum, and then the hapten is administered. Being small, the hapten quickly clears from the body, but before this occurs, some of it enters the interstitial fluid space (ISFS) of the tumor and is captured by the hapten-specific Fab. Theoretically, very high lesion-to-background ratios are possible with this system. Furthermore, the kinetics are highly manipulable. Further studies are needed to determine the potential utility of this approach for RID.

In my opinion, at the present time, ^{111}In offers greater advantages than its competitors as a radionuclide for RID. This opinion is based on the isotope's overall characteristics and the fact that the patient can be followed with serial images for several days to see if a putative lesion remains at a specific site, thereby increasing the possibility of its being real. In fairness to those investigators who are working with ^{123}I and ^{99m}Tc, this technology is still in a developmental stage, and as advances are made, the arguments in favor of ^{111}In may change. If RID grows in importance, this issue may not be resolved for many years.

RELEVANCE OF BASIC TUMOR AND NORMAL TISSUE PHYSIOLOGY TO SUCCESSFUL RID

As noted previously, the antibody, while important for radioimmunodetection, is not the only important variable involved in successful tumor detection. Indeed, anatomical and physiological aspects of the tumor and normal tissues are probably more important to the absolute concentration of the radionuclide in these tissues than are the characteristics of the antibody. Regardless of the immunoreactive molecule administered, once it enters the vascular compartment it circulates through organs having a wide range of blood flows and sometimes dramatically different vascular architecture. The liver, for example, receives over 0.5 ml of blood per minute per gram of tissue and its sinusoids will allow penetration by very large molecules [63]. The gastrointestinal tract can have a very high blood flow (especially in the immediate postprandial state), and it too will admit relatively large molecules through its capillaries [64]. The kidney, which maintains tight integrity of its capillary endothelium, receives over 3 ml of blood per gram of tissue per minute [65]. Many organs receive a huge amount of blood in a very short period of time. Within some of these organs are receptor-bearing cells or other sites capable of acquiring and destroying proteins. Thus, the antibody or antibody fragment is in constant jeopardy of being removed from the vascular compartment and either excreted or destroyed.

As previously indicated, the pharmacodynamics of these effects can also vary from antibody to antibody. Consider the outcome if the injected antibody had a proclivity for the liver! It must also be remembered that these organs are large compared to the size of a primary neoplasm or metastatic site. A tumor the size of a baseball (about 2.8 in. in diameter) would be considered quite large. If it were shaped like a sphere, it would weigh approximately 188 g. That is just slightly more than the weight of one kidney in the average adult man (150 g) [66]. Since tumors only get about 0.2 ml of blood flow per gram of tumor per minute [67], the tumor would receive only 38 ml of blood each minute. *This scenario assumes a best-case situation for the tumor blood flow.* On the other hand, one kidney, which weighs 38 g less than the tumor, would receive 300 ml in that same minute, or 8 times as much as the tumor. The liver would receive over 700 ml each minute. Unfortunately for

RID, as tumors increase in size their blood flow on a per gram basis decreases. A tumor the size of a baseball may receive an order of magnitude less than 0.2 ml per gram of tumor per minute [67–73], and for a variety of reasons the distribution of that blood flow will vary considerably in different parts of the tumor. Much of the blood may not even perfuse the tumor due to arteriovenous shunting [71]. Thus, low tumor blood flow and high normal organ blood flow can, and does, cause great problems in RID. Given the tumor blood flow problem, it is easy to see how even a small drop in the quantity of labeled antibody remaining in the vascular compartment can significantly reduce the absolute tracer concentration within the lesion.

In those lesions where the tumor is small and the blood flow relatively high, other problems arise to limit tumor concentration of the radiopharmaceutical. One barrier is the tumor capillary. Although it is true that large molecular weight proteins can penetrate a tumor capillary more easily than a renal capillary (owing to the architectural disturbance inherent in capillaries born in malignant tissue) [72], the tumor capillary still appears to be a deterrent to the passage of the radiopharmaceutical into the tumor's ISFS [73]. In cases where the capillaries have good integrity, a very small percentage of the high-molecular-weight proteins actually crosses into the tumor ISFS. Those antibodies that do cross into the interstitium of the tumor must make their way to the tumor cells. In contrast to small molecules, which are readily diffusible, high-molecular-weight proteins travel through tissue ISFS by convection currents. The radiolabeled antibody moves ponderously between the tumor cells, generally attaching to those cells nearest the capillary endothelium. Autoradiographs by Mach and others have shown that the larger the immunoreactive molecule, the shorter its migration distance from the capillary wall [74]. Thus, the Fab' fragment can be expected to go deeper into the tumor than the F(ab')2, which will, in turn, go deeper into the tumor than the intact antibody molecule.

It will not make any difference how far the molecule penetrates the tumor tissue, however, if it does not find an antigen. When one examines a variety of lesions, it becomes obvious that some sections of the tumor can be totally devoid of antigen while other parts have an abundance. If there is no antigen present to bind the radiolabeled antibody, it is in jeopardy of being swept from the tumor by the very currents that carried it to the tumor cell. Furthermore, in the case of certain antigens, it is entirely possible (but not proven) that immune complexes are shed and leave the tumor. In other ways, however, the tumor actually helps to retain a radiolabeled antibody. The venous outflow of tumors is poor, beginning with the venules themselves. As the tumors enlarge, the architecture of the venule becomes steadily more chaotic until a near stagnation occurs. Further, there are no lymphatics in tumors, so egress by that route is not feasible. Even nonspecific antibodies will concentrate in tumor tissue to some degree. The molecules are probably trapped in the tumor mass and in some way internalized by its cells.

Based on the tumor physiology as described, it appears that fragments of antibody (provided they remain attached to the available antigen) should be the best form of immunoreactive molecule for RID. Indeed, when the kidneys of tumor-bearing nude mice were tied off, twice as much ^{111}In was acquired by the tumor after administration of [111]In Fab' compared with administration of the labeled intact antibody [75]. Nonetheless, small molecules such as Fab can be eliminated through, or acquired by, the kidney [76]. Fab also enters other tissues more easily. The end result is that the blood levels of [111]In Fab fall rapidly [60], and therefore, one accumulates less of the Fab and F(ab')2 fragments in the tumor than the accumulation that occurs with intact antibody. Thus, for absolute concentration in a tumor, the best immunoreactive molecule to use is the intact form. However, the lesion-to-background ratios compatible with effective imaging are achieved much faster and are higher for the fragments than for the intact antibody molecule.

A LOOK TO THE FUTURE

There is no question that radiolabeled antibodies can detect lesions in some tumor systems that are missed by the standard techniques such as computed tomography, ultrasound, or magnetic resonance imaging [52,78]. It is equally true that we are dealing with a modality that is far from optimal. RID is a hard system to optimize. The animal models used to develop the concepts to be taken into humans have not proven as useful in this technology as they have in other branches of radiopharmaceutical development. As a consequence, a great deal of time has been devoted to basic science programs that have had limited value when the concept was carried to human subjects. At present we face the limitations that intact antibodies produce images with high background and that they require a delay of several days between administration and optimal imaging. Further, the large molecule is a strong inducer of human antimouse antibodies (HAMA), and HAMA could make a second administration of the antibody potentially dangerous or could possibly lead to image degradation due to rapid hepatic clearance of the immunoconjugate. Recent evidence, however, does indicate that imaging can be performed in the face of HAMA with worthwhile results [79].

The first and most obvious option for change is the use of small fragments. These can be produced using standard digestion techniques; however, the production of a stable F(ab')2 is not easy. Some monoclonal antibodies produce F(ab')2 fragments that have a reasonable degree of stability. Others produce highly unstable molecules that reduce to the smaller Fab' [61]. If fragments can be prepared successfully, however, the end result should be an improvement in imaging with a modest reduction in background. Specifically, lesions in the liver and mediastinum should become more obvious, especially with the use of SPECT imaging.

The production of engineered antibodies, the so-called chimeric antibodies, could reduce the HAMA problem. This might prove to be a significant advance if repeated administration of these products is desired. While great things are predicted for the chimeric antibodies, they must still face problems of tumor physiology. Theoretically, tumor targeting with chimerics will not be greatly improved over that achieved with murine IgG.

Alterations of the isoelectric point of the antibody molecule might change its distribution in the body. By this approach, it might be possible to reduce the uptake of Fab' fragments by the kidneys [80]. This would, in turn, reduce the radiation dose to that organ. The key issue, however, will be whether this approach can be used without loss of immunoreactivity (affinity?). Work in our laboratory has suggested that this approach can successfully reduce the renal uptake of a Fab. Unfortunately, we have been unable to accomplish this without a 50% reduction in immunoreactivity and/or affinity.

As for human monoclonal antibodies, they tend to be of low affinity. Theoretically, low-affinity antibodies should not work as well as high-affinity antibodies. However, the need for increased affinity for effective RID is yet to be determined. Human antibodies would reduce the production of HAMA, and it is possible that they might have a more favorable distribution in humans than murine antibodies. However, clinical trials will have to be performed to demonstrate these potential advantages. Presently, human monoclonal IgGs with "acceptable" affinity are not easy to make and have yet to become a number one priority for RID. In addition, the expected longer half-life of human or humanized antibodies should lead to increased duration of blood pool activity, which could limit the use of these reagents for RID.

Finally, exotic mechanisms such as the "hapten" system could be significant for RID. Clinical trials have been performed using the hapten system, and some encouraging results have been developed [81].

What precisely do we wish to accomplish with RID? Given the philosophy of medical practice today, most physicians would agree

1. that it would be worthwhile under certain circumstances for the detection of metastatic lesions;
2. that we should be able to use RID safely;
3. that we should be able to follow the patient's progress by RID as long as clinically desirable.

Given these potential use criteria, what is the smallest lesion we wish to see? How good should we try to get? In many cases, the early diagnosis of widely metastatic disease is not of benefit. One could utilize currently available RID systems. However, this is an era of exponential advancement in bioscience, and one is ill advised to prepare only for the moment. RID research, in the opinion of the author, should continue to be directed toward providing the best detection system possible.

REFERENCES

1. Pressman D, Korngold L. The in vivo localization of anti-Wagner osteogenic sarcoma antibodies. Cancer 1953; 6:619–23.
2. Korngold L, Pressman D. The localization of antilymphosarcoma antibodies in the Murphy lymphosarcoma of the rat. Cancer Res 1954; 14:96–9.
3. Fudenberg HH, Pink GRL, Wang A-C, Ferrara GB, eds. Basic immunogenetics. 3rd ed. Oxford: Oxford University Press, 1984.
4. Kline J, ed. Immunology: the science of self–non-self discrimination. New York: Wiley, 1982.
5. Halpern SE, Hagan PL, Chen A. Distribution of radiolabeled human and mouse monoclonal IgM antibodies in murine models. J Nucl Med 1988; 29:1688–96.
6. Ryan KP, Dillman RO, DeNardo SJ, et al. Breast cancer imaging with In–111 human IgM monoclonal antibodies: preliminary studies. Radiology 1988; 167:71–5.
7. Rennke HG, Venkatachalam MA. Glomerular permeability: in vivo tracer studies with polyanionic and polycationic ferritins. Kidney Int 1977; 11:44–53.
8. Brenner BM, Hostetler TH, Humes HD. Glomerular permeability: barrier function based on discrimination of molecular size and charge. Am J. Physiol 1978; 234:455–60.
9. Rennke HG, Patel Y, Venkatachalam MA. Glomerular filtration of proteins: clearance of anionic, neutral and cationic horseradish peroxidase in the rat. Kidney Int 1978; 13:278–88.
10. Halpern SE, Dillman RO. Problems associated with radioimmunodetection and possibilities for future solutions. J Biol Resp Mod 1987; 6:235–62.
11. Halpern SE, Hagan P, Garver P, et al. Stability, characterization, and kinetics of 111 In-labeled monoclonal antitumor antibodies in normal animals and nude mouse – human tumor models. Cancer Res 1983; 43:5347–55.
12. Kohler GP, Milstein C. Continuous cultures of fused cells secreting antibody of predetermined specificity. Nature 1975; 256:495–7.
13. Paul WE, ed. Fundamental immunology. New York: Raven Press, 1984; 751–6.
14. Potter M. Immunoglobulin-producing tumors. In: Myeloma proteins of mice. Physiol Rev 1972; 52:631.
15. Potter M. Antigen-binding myeloma proteins of mice. In: Kunkel HG, Dixon FJ, eds. Adv Immunol. Orlando: Academic Press; 1977; 25:141–211.
16. Barski G, Soriceal S, Cornefert F. "Hybrid" type cells in combined cultures of two different mammalian cell strains. J Natl Cancer Inst 1961; 26:1269.

18. Pontevarco G. Production of indefinitely multiplying mammalian cellmatic cell hybrids by polyethylene glycol "PEG" treatment. Somat Cell Genet 1976; 1:397.

19. Bale WF, Contreras MA, Izzo MJ, et al. Preferential in vivo localization of 125 I-labeled antibody in a carcinogen induced syngeneic rat tumor. Prog Exp Tumor Res 1974; 19:270–83.

20. Goldenberg DM, Preston, DF, Primus FC, et al. Photoscan localization of G.W.-39 tumors in hamsters using radiolabeled anticarcinoembryonic antigen immunoglobulin G. Cancer Res 1974; 34:1–9.

21. Hoffer PB, Lathrop K, Bekerman C. Use of 131 I-CEA antibody as a tumor scanning agent. J Nucl Med 1974; 15:323–7.

22. Primus FJ, Wang RH, Goldenberg DM, et al. Localization of human GW-39 tumors in hamsters by radiolabeled heterospecific antibody to carcinoembryonic antigen. Cancer Res 1973; 33:2977–83.

23. Mach JP, Carrel S, Merenda C, et al. In vivo localization of radiolabeled antibodies to carcinoembryonic antigen in human carcinoma grafted into nude mice. Nature 1974; 248:704–6.

24. Hagan PL, Halpern SE, Dillman RO, et al. Tumor size; effect on monoclonal antibody uptake in tumor models. J Nucl Med 1986; 27:422–7.

25. Goldenberg DN, DeLand FH, Kim E, et al. Use of radiolabeled antibodies to carcinoembryonic antigen for the detection and localization of diverse cancers by external photo scanning. N Engl J Med 1978; 298:1384–8.

26. Mach JP, Carrel S, Forni N, et al. Tumor localization of radiolabeled antibodies against carcinoembryonic antigen in patients with carcinoma. N Engl J Med 1980; 303:5–10.

27. Mach JP, Buchegger F, Forni N, et al. Use of radiolabeled monoclonal anti-CEA antibodies for the detection of human carcinomas by external photo scanning and tomoscintigraphy. Immunol Today 1981; 2:239–49.

28. Larson SM, Brown JP, Wright PW, Carrasquillo JA, et al. Imaging of melanoma with I-131-labeled monoclonal antibodies. J Nucl Med 1983; 24:123–9.

29. Britton K, Granowska M. Experience with I-123 labeled antibodies. In: Srivastava SC, ed. New York and London: Plenum Press, 1988:177–91.

30. Larson S, Carrasquillo JA, Reynolds J. The NIH experience with radiolabeled monoclonal antibodies: lymphoma, melanoma, and colon cancer. In: Srivastava, SC, ed. New York and London: Plenum Press, 1988:393–407.

31. Mach JP, Buchegger F, Bischof-Delaloye A, et al. Progress in diagnostic immunoscintigraphy and the first approach to radioimmunotherapy of colon carcinoma. In: Srivastava SC, ed. Radiolabeled monoclonal antibodies for imaging and therapy. New York and London: Plenum Press, 1988:95–110.

32. Delaloye B, Bischof-Delaloye A, Buchegger F, et al. Detection of colorectal carcinoma by emission-computerized tomography after injection of I-123-labeled FAB or F(ab')2 fragments from monoclonal anti-carcinoembryonic antigen antibodies. J Clin Invest 1986; 77:301–11.

33. David GS, Reisfield RA. Protein iodination with solid state lactoperoxidase. Biochemistry 1974; 13:1014.

34. Hunter WM, Greenwood C. Preparation of I-131 labeled human growth hormone of high specific activity. Nature 1982; 194:495.

35. Wilbur DS, Jones DS, Fritzberg AR, et al. Radioiodination of monoclonal antibodies. Labeling with *para*-iodophenyl (PIP) derivatives for in vivo stability of the radioiodine label. J Nucl Med 1986; 27:959.

36. Stern P, Hagan PL, Halpern SE, et al. The effect of the radiolabel on the kinetics of monoclonal anti-CEA in a nude mouse – human colon tumor model. In: Mitchell MS, Oettgen HF, eds. Hybridomas in cancer diagnosis and treatment. New York: Raven Press, 1982.

37. Halpern SE, Stern PH, Hagan PL, et al. The labeling of monoclonal antibodies with 111-In: technique and advantages compared to radioiodine labeling. In: Burchial SW, Rhodes BA, eds. Radioimmunoimaging and radioimmunotherapy. New York: Elsevier, 1983:197–205.

38. Halpern SE, Dillman RO, Hagan PL. Problems and promise of monoclonal anti-tumor antibodies. Diagnostic Imaging 1983; 40–7.

39. Zalutsky MR. Radiohalogenation of antibodies: chemical aspects. In: Srivastava SC, ed. Radiolabeled monoclonal antibodies for imaging and therapy. New York and London: Plenum Press, 1988:195–213.

40. Halpern SE. The advantages and limits of In-111 labeling of antibodies: experimental studies and clinical applications. Nucl Med Biol 1986; 13:195–210.

41. Halpern SE, Hagan PL, Garver PR. Comparison of In-111 anti-CEA monoclonal antibodies (MoAb) and endogenously labeled Se-75 MoAb's in normal and tumor-bearing mice. J Nucl Med 1982; 23:8.

42. Sundberg MW, Mears CF, Goodwin DA, et al. Chelating agents for the binding of metal ions to macromolecules. Nature 1974; 256:587.

43. Meares CF, McCall MJ, Reardon DT, et al. Conjugation of antibodies with bifunctional chelating agents azothiocyanate and bromacetamide reagents: methods of analysis, and subsequent addition of metal ions. Anal Biochem 1984; 142:68–78.

44. Krejcarek GE, Tucker KL. Covalent attachment of chelating groups to macromolecules. Biochem Biophys Res Commun 1977; 77:581–5.

45. Esteban JM, Schlom J, Gansow OA, et al. New method for the chelation of In-111 to monoclonal antibodies: biodistribution and imaging of athymic mice bearing human colon carcinoma xenografts. J Nucl Med 1987; 28:861–70.

46. Unpublished data of the author.

47. Wilkening D, Srinivasan A, Kasina S, et al. Tc-99m antibody labeling with N3S and N2S2 amide mercaptides: active ester complex yield and side chain length. J Nucl Med 1988; 29:815.

48. Rao TN, Vanderheyden J-L, Kasina S, et al. Dependence of immunoreactivity and tumor uptake on ratio of Tc and Re N2S2 complexes for antibody Fab fragment. J Nucl Med 1988; 29:815.

49. Simonson RB, Ultee ME, Houston FM, et al. Imaging of tumor xenografts with monoclonal antibodies labeled at their carbohydrate residues with technetium-99m. J Nucl Med 1988; 29:815.

50. Wahl RL, Johnson J, Mallette S, et al. Clinical experience with Tc-99m anti-melanoma fragments and SPECT. J Nucl Med 1988; 29:812.

51. Fer MF, Schroff RW, Abrams PG, et al. Successful imaging of lung and colon carcinomas by a Tc-99m labeled monoclonal antibody. J Nucl Med 1988; 29:834.

52. Baum RP, Lorenz M, Hottenrott C, et al. Immunoscintigraphy of known and occult metastatic colorectal carcinoma with Tc-99m anti-CEA monoclonal antibody. J Nucl Med 1988; 29:834.
53. Halpern SE, Dillman RO, Witztum KF, et al. Radioimmunodetection of melanoma using In-111 96.5 monoclonal antibody: a preliminary report. Radiology 1985; 155:493–9.
54. Halpern SE, Haindl W, Beauregard J, et al. Scintigraphy with In-111-labeled monoclonal anti-tumor antibodies: kinetics, biodistribution and tumor detection. Radiology 1988; 168:529–36.
55. Halpern SE, Dillman RO. Use of radiolabeled antibodies in diagnosis and staging of solid tumors. In: Pattengale PK, Lukes RJ, Taylor CR, eds. Lymphoproliferative diseases: pathogenesis, diagnosis, therapy. New York: Martinus Nijhof, 1984.
56. Carrasquillo JA, Bonn PA, Keenan AM, et al. Radioimmunodetection of cutaneous T-cell lymphoma with 111-In-labeled T-101 monoclonal antibody. N Engl J Med 1986; 315:673–80.
57. Abdel-Nabi HH, Schwartz AN, Higgano CS, et al. Colorectal carcinoma: detection with In-111 anti-carcinoembryonic-antigen monoclonal antibody ZCE-025. Radiology 1987; 164:617–21.
58. Lamki LM, Patt YZ, Murray JL, et al. The role of 111-In anti-CEA monoclonal antibodies in the detection of occult metastatic cancer in patients with rising serum CEA. J Nucl Med 1988; 29:833–4.
59. Halpern SE. Personal observations of the author.
60. Halpern SE, Carroll RG, Tarbutron JP. Imaging (I) with 111-In Fab' of an anti-CEA antibody (A): comparison with its 111-In intact and F(ab')2 derivative (D). J Nucl Med 1988;29:812.
61. Halpern SE, Hagan PL, Bartholomew RM. The distribution of various 111-In F(ab')2 preparations in normal mice, J Nucl Med 1987; 28:692.
62. Frincke JM, Halpern SE, Chang CH, et al. Radioimmunodetection (RID) approach using a 111-In hapten (H) monoclonal antibody (MoAb): studies in the nude mouse–human colon tumor model. J Nucl Med 1987; 28:711.
63. Guyton AC. Textbook of medical physiology. Philadelphia: Saunders, 1986:836.
64. Guyton AC. Textbook of medical physiology. Philadelphia: Saunders, 1986:342.
65. Brenner BM, Zatz R, Ichikawa L. The renal circulations. In: Brenner BM, Rector FC, eds. The Kidney. 3rd ed. Philadelphia: Saunders, 1985:93.
66. Tisher CC, Madsen KM. Anatomy of the Kidney. In: Brenner BM, Rector FC, eds. The kidney. 3rd ed. Philadelphia: Saunders, 1986:3.
67. Guillino P, Grantham F. Studies on the exchange of the fluids between host and tumor. II. The blood flow of hepatomas and other tumors in rats and mice. J Natl Cancer Inst 1961; 27:1465–84.
68. Tannock I. Population kinetics of carcinoma cells, capillary endothelial cells, and fibroblasts in a transplanted mouse mammary tumor. Cancer Res 1970; 30:2470–6.
69. Tannock I, Steel G. Quantitative techniques for study of the anatomy and function of small blood vessels in tumors. J Natl Cancer Inst 1969; 42:771–82.

70. Vaupel P. Interrelation between mean arterial blood pressure, blood flow and vascular resistance in solid tumor tissue of DS-carcinosarcoma. Experientia 1975; 3:587–9.

71. Vaupel P, Grunewald W, Manz R, et al. Intercapillary HbO2 saturation in tumor tissue of DS-carcinosarcoma during normoxia. In: Silver I, Erecinska M, Bicher H, eds. Oxygen transport to tissue–III. New York: Plenum Press, 1978.

72. Warren B. The ultra structure of the microcirculation at the advancing edge of Walker 256 carcinoma. Microvasc Res 1970; 2:443–53.

73. Peterson HL, Appelgren L, Kjartansson I. Tumor blood flow and tumor vessel permeability. Bibl Anat 1977; 15:277–80.

74. Buchegger F, Haskell CM, Schreyer M, et al. Radiolabeled fragments of monoclonal anti-CEA antibodies for localization of human colon carcinoma grafted into nude mice. J Exp Med 1983; 158:413–27.

75. Halpern S, Buchegger F, Schreyer M, et al. Effect of size of radiolabeled antibody and fragments on tumor uptake and distribution in nephrectomized mice. J Nucl Med 1984; 25:112.

76. Sumpio BE, Maack T. Kinetics, competition and selectivity of tubular absorption of proteins. Am J Physiol 1982; 243:F379–92.

77. Halpern S, Carroll RG, Tarburton JP, et al. Imaging (I) with 111-In Fab' of an anti-CEA antibody (A): comparison with its 111-In intact and F(ab')2 derivative (D). J Nucl Med 1988; 29:812.

78. Halpern SE, Amox DG, Eakin DA, et al. Utility of 111In-labeled monoclonal antibodies (111In MoAb) in detection (D) of occult metastasis (M). J Nucl Med 1988; 29:893.

79. Abdel-Nabi H, Doerr R, Roth SC, et al. Recurrent colorectal carcinoma detection with repeated infusions of In-111 ZCE-025 MoAb. J Nucl Med 1989; 30:748.

80. Tarburton JP, Halpern SE, Hagan P, et al. Effect of acetylation on monoclonal antibody ZCE-025 Fab': distribution in normal and tumor bearing mice. J Biol Resp Mod 1990; 9:221–30.

81. Slater JB, Frincke JM, Stickney OR. The role of CEA as a metabolic indicator to predict the pharmacokinetics of the bifunctional antibody system (BFA) in colon carcinoma. J Nucl Med 1989; 30:905.

2

Generation and Characterization of Monoclonal Antibody B72.3

Experimental and Preclinical Studies

David M. Colcher,* Diane E. Milenic, and Jeffrey Schlom

National Cancer Institute, National Institutes of Health
Bethesda, Maryland

INTRODUCTION

Monoclonal antibodies (MAb) have had a great impact in the field of tumor immunology and have provided the impetus to many of the recent advances made in this area. MAbs have made it possible for investigators to identify and characterize tumor-associated antigens (TAA) that were previously unknown or, at best, poorly defined. One area of great potential for MAbs generated against tumor-associated antigens is in the management of cancer patients. Applications in this area range from diagnosis of disease to the treatment of patients.

The rationale for the generation of many of the monoclonal antibodies made by this laboratory, including MAb B72.3, was to utilize tissue extracts of metastatic carcinomas as immunogens in an attempt to generate monoclonal antibodies reactive with antigenic determinants present in metastatic lesions, which are the clinically important lesions in the management of malignancies. The primary tumor may not express the relevant antigens to the extent found on the metastatic lesion. Additionally, the selective pressures exerted in the establishment of a cell line may modify or eliminate some antigens present in the original tumor tissue. This has proven to be the case with the B72.3-reactive antigen TAG-72, as discussed below.

*Present affiliation: University of Nebraska Medical Center, Omaha, Nebraska.

MAb B72.3 was generated by immunizing BALB/c mice with a membrane-enriched fraction of a human mammary carcinoma metastasis to the liver. Multiple assays using tumor and normal tissue extracts, live cells in culture, and tissue sections were employed to determine the specificity of MAb B72.3 [1,2].

DISTRIBUTION OF TAG-72 EXPRESSION

MAb B72.3 has been tested against a spectrum of adult and fetal tissues using avidin-biotin complex immunohistochemical techniques to evaluate the expression of the reactive TAG-72 antigen [2–5]. TAG-72 has been shown to be expressed in several epithelial-derived malignancies, including the vast majority of colonic adenocarcinomas, invasive ductal carcinomas of the breast, non–small cell lung carcinomas, common epithelial histological types of ovarian carcinomas, as well as the majority of pancreatic, gastric, and esophageal cancers evaluated. Using the optimal MAb B72.3 incubation conditions (2mg/ml, overnight at 4°C), a variety of formalin-fixed, paraffin-embedded human tumors were analyzed for expression of TAG-72 (Table 1). Adenocarcinomas demonstrated the most TAG-72 expression, with 100% of ovarian (40 of 40) and endometrial (32 of 32), 96% (32 of 33) of lung, 94% (51 of 54) of colon, 84% (37 of 44) of breast, 88% (23 of 26) of pancreatic, and 88% (35 of 40) of gastric tumors expressing TAG-72 on some tumor cells. Of these, ovarian, colonic, lung, and breast adenocarcinomas demonstrated the highest average percentage of cellular reactivities. Squamous cell carcinomas demonstrated variable reactivity with MAb B72.3, and poorly differentiated squamous cell carcinomas often showed more TAG-72 antigen expression than well-differentiated keratin-producing tumors from the same primary organs (lung, esophagus).

At least 5% of the malignant epithelial cells were positive in the majority of adenocarcinomas of the breast, colon, lung, pancreas, stomach, and ovary as well as esophageal squamous carcinomas. TAG-72 expression has not been detected, however, in tumors of neural, hemopoietic, or sarcomatous derivation, suggesting that the TAG-72 antigen is "pancarcinoma" in nature. No MAb B72.3 reactivity, or only trace amounts, has been observed with a wide range of adult normal tissues, with limited reactivity noted in a few benign tissues, such as breast and colon as well as transitional epithelium [4,6]. TAG-72 has been shown to be expressed at high levels in secretory endometrium; it is not found, however, in resting or postmenopausal endometrium [7]. TAG-72 antigen expression has been detected, however, in fetal colon, stomach, and esophagus, thus also defining TAG-72 as an oncofetal antigen [4]. TAG-72 has also been shown to be distinct from other tumor-associated antigens (see below).

Table 1 B72.3 Reactivity with Human Malignancies

		Reactive lesions[a]	
Organ	Histological type	>5%[b]	>20%[b]
Ovary	Serous cystadenocarcinoma	30/30	14/30
	Mucinous cystadenocarcinoma	10/10	6/10
Lung	Non–small cell carcinoma	32/33	21/33
	Small cell carcinoma	0/18	0/18
Colon	Adenocarcinoma	51/54	23/54
Gastric	Adenocarcinoma	35/40	25/40
Pancreatic	Adenocarcinoma	23/26	13/26
Breast	Invasive ductal carcinoma	37/44	12/44
Endometrium	Adenocarcinoma	32/32	27/32
Miscellaneous	Nonepithelial malignancies	0/10	0/10

[a]Number reactive/number evaluated.
[b]Percentage of cells reactive with B72.3 using fixed sections and the avidin-biotin immunohistochemistry methodology.
Source: Data taken from Refs. 2,3,43,44

TAG-72 EXPRESSION IN CELL LINES VERSUS TUMORS

While TAG-72 is expressed in the majority of adenocarcinomas, only 1 of 25 breast cancer cell lines [MCF-7 (one variant)] and 1 of 18 colon cancer cell lines (LS-174T) express this antigen at detectable levels [8]. Furthermore, TAG-72 expression in these two cell lines was shown to be a property of a low percentage of cells within each culture. This phenomenon has been further analyzed by examining the extent of antigenic modulation of human mammary tumor cell populations, via the temporal analyses of cloned MCF-7 mammary tumor cell populations [8].

Environmental milieu and the three-dimensional configuration of tumor masses have also been shown to play a role in modulating tumor antigen expression. A study by Friedman et al. [9] demonstrated that levels of cell surface TAG-72 diminished within days after the primary colon carcinomas were placed in cell culture; in contrast, carcinoembryonic antigen (CEA) levels remained constant after establishment of the cultures. An increase in TAG-72 expression was observed, moreover, when the LS-174T colon carcinoma cells were grown under culture conditions that promote three-dimensional growth [10]. LS-174T cells grown in spheroid or suspension cultures demonstrated a two- to seven-fold increase in TAG-72 antigen expression, while those grown on agar plugs demonstrated a 10-fold increase. When the LS–174T cell line was injected into athymic mice to generate tumors, the level of TAG–72

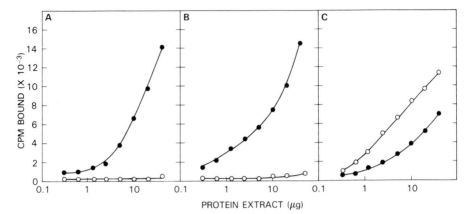

Figure 1 Expression of TAG-72 (using MAb B72.3) and carcinoembryonic antigen (CEA) (using MAb B1.1) in LS-174T cells grown in culture and as tumors in athymic mice. Approximately 4 ng of ^{125}I-B72.3 was added to increasing amounts of protein extracts (A) of a human breast tumor metastasis to the liver (●) and to normal human liver (○); (B) LS-174T cells grown in culture (○) and as a tumor in athymic mice (●); (C) ^{125}I-B1.1 (approximately 2 ng), a MAb reactive with CEA that was used in a solid-phase RIA with increasing amounts of protein extracts of LS-174T cells grown as a tumor in athymic mice (●) or LS-174T cells grown in monolayer culture (○). (From Horan Hand et al. [10]).

increased over 100-fold, to levels compared to those seen in tumor masses from patients (Fig. 1).

The latter two studies [9,10] help to explain the phenomenon in which the TAG-72 determinant is absent in virtually all carcinoma cell lines examined but is present in the vast majority of carcinoma biopsies. Thus, the variability of expression of TAAs, via either antigenic heterogeneity or antigenic modulation, presents a potential problem in the development and optimization of immunodiagnostic and/or immunotherapeutic procedures for carcinomas.

AUGMENTATION OF TUMOR ANTIGEN EXPRESSION

One approach to the problem of antigenic modulation is the use of biological response modifiers to enhance the expression of tumor antigens on the surface of carcinoma cells. The treatment of human breast or colon carcinoma cells with recombinant human leukocyte interferon (IFN)- α A has been shown to increase the surface expression of specific TAAs recognized by MAbs [11,12]. The binding of the MAbs to the surface of tumor cells increased in a dose-dependent manner, with optimal levels of TAA enhancement of 100–1000 units of IFN-αA/ml; higher concentrations of IFN-αA, which were cytostatic or cytotoxic, were less effective in enhancing TAA expression. The ability of recombinant IFN- αA to increase the expression of TAAs on human carcinoma cells showed temporal dependency, with optimal enhancement occurring after 16–24 hr. It has also been demonstrated [11,12] that the IFN-αA-mediated increase in surface antigen is a result of both accumulation of more antigen per cell and an increase in the percentage of cells expressing the antigen. It has also been demonstrated that IFN-γ can similarly mediate the up-regulation of tumor antigen expression [13].

These studies have been extended to analyze the ability of interferons to enhance TAG-72 expression on freshly isolated tumor cells [14]. Cells were isolated from patients with pleural or peritoneal effusions and cytologically diagnosed as adenocarcinoma (n = 43), malignant nonepithelial neoplasms (n = 10), or benign lesions (n = 8). Both type I and II IFNs enhanced the expression of TAG-72 and altered the level of expression of the major histocompatibility antigens. Comparative studies of three different human IFNs (IFN-αA, IFN-β_{ser}, and IFN-γ) revealed that IFN-γ was the most potent in augmenting B72.3 binding (Fig. 2A–D). Unlike the IFN-γ-mediated induction of the class II human leukocyte antigens, the change in tumor antigen expression consisted of enhanced constitutive antigen expression; de novo induction of TAG-72 could not be achieved by either type I or type II IFN (Fig. 2E,F). Of 43 effusions isolated from different adenocarcinoma patients, 35 (81%) expressed TAG-72. Treatment with Hu-IFN increased the level of expression of TAG-72 in 27 of 35 samples (77.1%). These studies demonstrate the augmentation of tumor-associated antigens by Hu-IFNs and indicate that these biological response modifiers may be used to enhance the binding of conjugated MAbs to freshly isolated human carcinoma cells.

CHARACTERIZATION OF THE TAG-72 ANTIGEN

The TAG-72 antigen has been purified from a human colon carcinoma xenograft, designated LS-174T, for further characterization [15]. The tumor homogenate was first fractionated by Sepharose CL-4B chromatography. The high-molecular-weight TAG-72 found in the exclusion volume was then subjected to two sequential passages through B72.3 antibody affinity columns. At each step of the procedure, the TAG-72 content was quantitated using a competition radioimmunoassay (RIA) [16]. The three-step procedure produced a purification of TAG-72 with minimal contamination by other proteins, as shown by polyacrylamide gel electrophoresis (PAGE), followed by staining with Coomassie blue or periodic acid/Schiff reagent. The density of affinity-purified TAG-72, as determined by cesium chloride gradient ultracentrifugation, was found to be

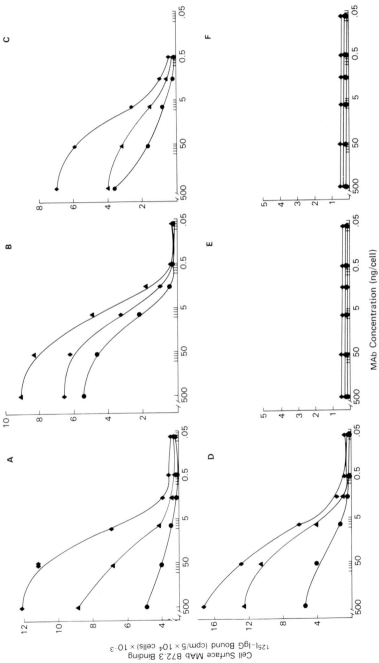

1.45 g/ml. This density determination, together with the high molecular weight of TAG-72, its resistance to chondroitinase digestion, the presence of blood-group-related oligosaccharides, and its sensitivity to shearing into lower-molecular-weight forms, suggest that TAG-72 is a mucin-like molecule. The apparent molecular weight of TAG-72, as determined by SDS-PAGE and Western blotting analyses, is greater than 10^6 daltons [15].

More recent studies, using a new series of MAbs generated against purified TAG-72 [17], have resulted in an over 1000-fold purification of TAG-72, permitting additional biochemical analyses [18]. These studies further demonstrated that TAG-72, with approximately 57% of the protein composition consisting of threonine, serine, proline, glycine, and alanine, is a mucin-like molecule because of the low amounts of methionine, tyrosine, and phenylalanine found in the purified TAG-72. Comparisons of the TAG-72 isolated from malignant effusions from four different carcinoma types have also been performed. These studies demonstrated similar biochemical and immunological properties among all the TAG-72 preparations (Fig. 3) [19].

SERUM ASSAYS FOR TAG-72

A major potential use of MAbs will be to detect specific carcinoma-associated antigens in sera of asymptomatic individuals and to indicate the presence of occult metastatic lesions in patients whose primary carcinoma has been previously excised. A competitive RIA for the detection of TAG-72 in tissue extracts and serum has been developed [16]. Serum from apparently healthy individuals contained an average of 2.2 U/ml of TAG-72, while 35% of carcinoma patients had elevated levels of serum TAG-72.

A double-determinant RIA for the detection of TAG-72 was subsequently developed to quantitate serum levels of the antigen [20]. In this assay, B72.3 was bound to a solid-phase matrix, and serum and ^{125}I-B72.3 were added. This simultaneous assay was somewhat easier to run and thus allowed the analysis of a large panel of serum samples. Serum from healthy blood donors

---

Figure 2 Relative ability of human interferon (Hu-IFN) - α A and Hu-IFN- γ to increase TAG-72 expression on the surface of human tumor cells isolated from serous effusions. The cellular component was isolated from serous effusions of patients diagnosed with carcinoma of the breast (A), lung (B), uterus (C), pancreas (D), melanoma (E), and a nonmalignant reactive mesothelium (F) incubated alone ($\bullet$) or with 1000–2000 U of Hu-IFN- αA ($\blacktriangle$) or Hu-IFN-γ ($\blacklozenge$) for 72 hr. TAG-72 expression was measured by adding 0.03–500 ng of B72.3 IgG/10^5 cells, followed by addition of approximately 10^5 cpm of ^{125}I-labeled goat antimouse IgG. Each point on the antibody dilution curves represents the mean of triplicate samples. (From Guadagni et al. [14].)

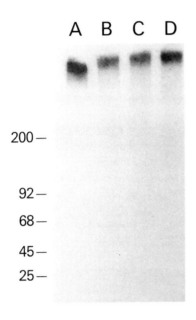

A B C D

200 —

92 —
68 —

45 —
25 —

Figure 3 Sodium dodecyl sulfate–polyacrylamide gel electrophoresis (SDS-PAGE) analysis of radioiodinated preparations of purified TAG-72. TAG-72 purified from patient effusions was radioiodinated, subjected to SDS-PAGE (3–12% gradient gel) under reducing conditions, and visualized by autoradiography. TAG-72 was purified from effusions of patients with carcinoma of ovary (A), colorectum (B), pancreas (C), and endometrium (D). (From Katari et al. [19].)

(1099 tested) had a mean TAG-72 level of 1.8 U/ml. Using a reference level of 10 U/ml, approximately 57% of patients with colorectal cancer exhibited elevated serum levels of TAG-72, whereas 1.3% of the healthy blood donors demonstrated similar elevations. Using a reference value of 20 U/ml, 37% of the colorectal cancer patient sera had elevated levels of TAG-72, while only 2 of the 1099 blood donor sera had similarly elevated values.

The TAG-72 antigen was purified and used to prepare a second generation of anti–TAG-72 MAbs. These MAbs were characterized as to their range of reactivities to tumor and normal tissues, using immunohistochemical techniques and RIAs, cell surface binding assays, and competitive RIAs, and as to their affinity constants (K_as) [17]. One of these MAbs, designated CC49, was shown to react with an epitope on TAG-72 that could be distinguished from that

Table 2   Summary of Serum TAG-72 Levels

Patient characteristics	Number of samples	Percentage with TAG-72 >6 U/ml
Carcinomas		
Esophagus	12	25
Gastric	291	40
Stage IV	93	57
Colorectal	177	43
Stages IV and V	74	60
Pancreas	13	31
Gallbladder	4	50
Choledochus	7	57
Lung	165	16
Adenocarcinoma	28	36
Squamous cell	60	17
Small cell	61	11
Non–small cell	16	19
Ovarian	97	26
Stage IV	15	53
Breast	118	16
Prostatic	50	20
Squamous	25	4
Sarcoma	29	3
Benign diseases		
Stomach	75	5
Colorectal	59	8
Miscellaneous	17	0
Normal	1258	2.5

Source: Data taken from Refs. 21-23.

recognized by B72.3. Moreover, while the K_a of B72.3 was shown to be 2.5 x 10^9 M^{-1}, that of CC49 was considerably higher (16.2 x 10^9 M^{-1}). These findings suggested that a more efficient assay for TAG-72 could be devised using both MAb CC49 and B72.3, with CC49 on a solid-phase matrix and ^{125}I-B72.3 as the detecting antibody. This combination enabled the development of a sequential assay (designated CA 72-4) for quantitating TAG-72 in biological fluids that showed optimal quantitative properties as demonstrated by such parameters as linear dose-response, high reproducibility, and lack of serum-matrix and "hookback" effects [21].

Only 2.5% of 1258 normal sera and 7.0% of 134 sera from patients with benign gastrointestinal diseases had TAG-72 levels greater than 6 U/ml in the CA 72-4 assay [21]. Approximately 40% of 504 patients with gastrointestinal malignancies had serum TAG-72 levels of greater than 6 U/ml (65% of the patients with advanced disease). Thirty-six percent of the patients with adenocarcinomas of the lung and 26% of patients with ovarian cancer (53% stage IV patients) also had elevated serum TAG-72 levels (Table 2).

A poor correlation was found between the CEA and TAG-72 values of sera obtained from gastric cancer patients. Thirty-seven percent of CEA-negative cases were scored positive in the CA 72-4 assay, suggesting the complementarity of the CA 72-4 assay to CEA assays in the analysis of sera from patients with certain malignancies [21–23].

PRECLINICAL ANALYSIS OF IODINATED B72.3 IgG

Initial studies were undertaken to evaluate the utility of labeled B72.3 IgG to localize human tumor tissue in situ. B72.3 IgG was purified using ion-exchange and size exclusion chromatography. The IgG was radiolabeled using Iodo-Gen without loss of immunoreactivity as long as an average of less than 1 mole of iodine per mole of IgG was used [24].

Radiolocalization studies were performed using athymic mice bearing colon carcinomas (LS-147T); a human melanoma xenograft (A375) was used as a TAG-72–negative control for nonspecific uptake of immunoglobulin. Seven to ten days after subcutaneous injection of the cells, when the tumors were approximately 0.3–0.5 cm in diameter, the mice were given intravenous injections of approximately 1.5 μCi of ^{125}I-B72.3 IgG (specific activity of $\approx$10 μCi/μg) or ^{125}I-MOPC-21 IgG (control antibody of the same isotype). The radiolocalization indices (RI), i.e., the percentage of the injected dose per gram (%ID/g), in the LS-174T tumor in comparison with that of various tissues were examined over a 7-day period. During this period, the RI rose, with tumor:liver, tumor:spleen, or tumor:kidney ratios reaching approximately 18:1 at day 7 (Fig. 4). Tumor:blood ratios also rose during this time, resulting in ratios of 5:1 at day 7. There was no specific uptake of ^{125}I-B72.3 IgG in any of the normal organs examined, including brain, muscle, stomach, intestines, uterus, and ovary. Approximately 10%ID/g reached the tumor 2 days after inoculation of the radiolabeled antibody. The amount of radiolabel at the tumor, as measured by the %ID/g, stayed constant over the first 4 days and then began to drop as the tumor increased in size. The total amount of activity in the

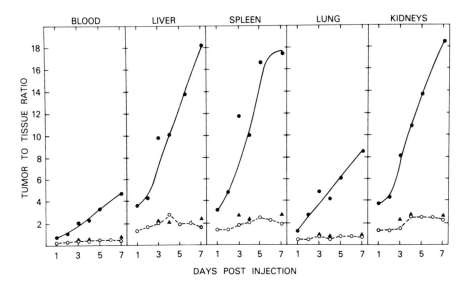

Figure 4 Tissue distribution of ^{125}I-B72.3 IgG in athymic mice bearing human tumors. Athymic mice bearing LS-174T colon carcinomas (●) or A375 melanomas (○) were inoculated with approximately 1.5 μCi of ^{125}I-B72.3 IgG. The mice were sacrificed over a 7-day period, and radioactivity per gram of tissue was determined. The ratio of the activity in the tumor as compared to other organs was plotted. Mice bearing LS-174T colon carcinomas were also injected with the control antibody MOPC-21 (▲). (From Colcher et al. [24].)

tumor stayed essentially constant over a 30-day period, while the activity in the rest of the body decreased significantly. The increased RIs resulted primarily from the clearance of labeled IgG from the blood pools.

Athymic mice bearing melanomas (A375, a TAG-72–negative tumor) were used as controls; no specific uptake of ^{125}I-B72.3 was observed in the tumors of these control animals. Similarly, no localization was observed in athymic mice bearing the colon carcinoma cell line when using ^{125}I-MOPC-21 IgG as a control antibody (Fig. 4). The same successful localization has been obtained more recently in clinical trials in patients with metastatic colorectal carcinomas (see following chapters).

RADIOIMMUNOTHERAPY USING IODINATED B72.3 IgG

The high degree of selective binding of B72.3 has led us to investigate its potential use as a radioimmunotherapeutic agent. The LS-174T xenograft, in which approximately 30–60% of tumor cells express TAG-72, was used to reflect the antigenic heterogeneity of TAG-72 often seen in patient biopsy specimens. Athymic mice bearing human colon carcinoma xenografts were injected with either 300 or 500 μCi of ^{131}I-B72.3 IgG to assess the effect of the radiolabeled MAb on the tumor growth as well as its potential side effects in vital organs [24]. In mice treated with the ^{131}I-B72.3 IgG, a marked inhibition of the growth of the human colon carcinoma xenografts was noticed in comparison with control mice injected with phosphate buffered saline (PBS) or control mice that received unlabeled B72.3 IgG. The tumors from these control mice weighed 2.7–3.7 times more than the tumors from the treated mice 17 days postinoculation of the radiolabeled MAb. Autoradiographic studies demonstrated a heterogeneous distribution of radioactivity throughout the tumor mass at 11 days postadministration of MAb. With time, the periphery of the tumor contained significantly less radioactivity than the medial areas, which were composed of predominantly nonviable tissue. These findings suggest that the more biologically active peripheral tumor zones, with higher mitotic rates, could have partially escaped the radiation effect of the single dose administered. The tumor cells may have continued dividing when the levels of circulating radiolabeled monoclonal antibody had decreased.

Toxicity was readily evident in the mice injected with the high-dose regimen (500 μCi), with confirmed bone marrow aplasia that proved lethal for 2 of 10 animals. The lower-dose regimen (300 μCi) resulted in bone marrow suppression of approximately 50% of the cells, which proved to be nonlethal. The tumors in the treated mice showed extensive necrosis caused by the lethal dose of ^{131}I-B72.3 that irreversibly damaged the cells. Radiation-induced terminal differentiation of cells was also found, as manifested by the drastically decreased mitotic count in treated animals (0–2 versus 12–14 per 10 high-power fields seen in control tumors).

Further studies were undertaken to determine whether multiple doses could reduce toxicity while effecting greater tumor cell death [26]. In contrast to a single 600-μCi dose of ^{131}I-B72.3 (Fig. 5A), where 50% of the animals died from toxicity, the administration of two 300-μCi doses of B72.3 (a total of 600 μCi) reduced or eliminated tumor growth in 90% of the mice, with only 10% of the animals dying from toxicity (Fig. 5B). Dose fractionation even permitted escalation of the dose to three 300-μCi doses (each 1 week apart) of B72.3 (for a total of 900 μCi) which resulted in even more efficient tumor reduction or elimination and minimal toxicity (Fig. 5C). The use of an isotype-matched control MAb revealed a nonspecific component to tumor growth retardation, but the use of the specific B72.3 demonstrated a much greater therapeutic effect. Tumors that had escaped MAb therapy were analyzed for expression of the B72.3-reactive TAG-72 antigen using the immunoperoxi-dase method and were shown to have the same antigenic phenotype as untreated tumors. Tumor elimination was verified by sacrificing the test animals follow–

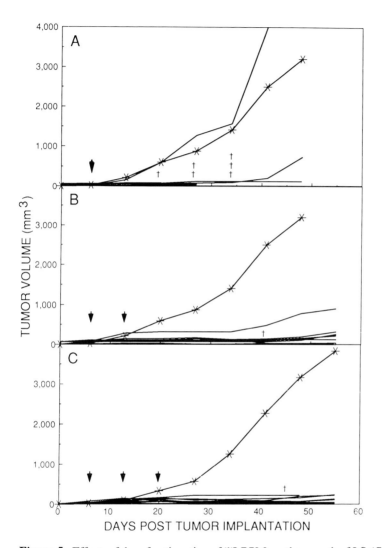

Figure 5 Effects of dose fractionation of ^{131}I-B72.3 on the growth of LS-174T colon carcinoma xenograft. The arrows denote the times of MAb administration, which began 7 days postadministration of LS-174T cells with 7-day intervals for animals receiving multiple doses of radiolabeled B72.3. Each line represents the tumor growth in an individual mouse. Asterisks represent the results obtained from mice receiving unlabeled B72.3 IgG ($n = 13$). A cross represents the death of a mouse. The doses administered were 600 μCi, once (A); 300 μCi, twice, for a total of 600 μCi (B); and 300 μCi, three times, for a total of 900 μCi (C). (Data from Schlom et al. [26].)

ing a 7 week observation period and performing histological examination of numerous organs including bone marrow. These studies demonstrated the advantage of dose fractionation of a radiolabeled MAb for tumor therapy.

PRECLINICAL ANALYSIS OF CHELATE-CONJUGATED B72.3 IgG

A wide spectrum of other radionuclides may be considered for use and may provide more efficient tumor eradication than iodine. Radionuclides that have such potential include ^{47}Sc, ^{67}Cu, ^{186}Re, and ^{188}Re, which emit both ß- and γ - rays; ^{90}Y, which is pure ß-emitter; as well as radionuclides that emit α - particles, such as ^{212}Pb, ^{212}Bi, and ^{211}At [27–29]. Labeling techniques using bifunctional chelates now permit proteins to be labeled with many of these radiometals. Chelating agents such as ethylenediaminetetraacetic acid (EDTA) and diethylenetriaminepentaacetic acid (DTPA) are most commonly used. The chelates themselves may be chemically modified to provide a method to link them to proteins. Examples are the cyclic and mixed anhydrides of DTPA [30,31]. Alternatively, linking groups may be incorporated in the chelate molecule by synthesis, as demonstrated by the use of the isothiocyanatobenzyl group (SCN-Bz) covalently linked to the carbon backbone of EDTA or DTPA [32,33].

Athymic mice bearing the LS-174T human colon carcinoma xenograft were injected with ^{111}In- or ^{88}Y-labeled (as a tracer for the potential use of ^{90}Y) B72.3 IgG that was modified using either the SCN-Bz-EDTA, CA-DTPA, or SCN-Bz-DTPA chelate conjugates [34]. Approximately 2.5 μCi of ^{111}In- or 0.5 μCi of ^{88}Y-labeled B72.3 IgG (0.05 metal ions/IgG molecule) was injected i.v. in mice bearing subcutaneous tumors. The mice were sacrificed at various times up to 7 days postinjection of the labeled MAb. At 48 hr, approximately 25%ID/g was found in the tumors of the mice injected with B72.3 IgG linked to both the SCN-Bz coupled chelates. This level stayed constant over the 7-day period of study. The mice injected with the ^{111}In-CA-DTPA-B72.3 localized approximately 19%ID/g in the tumor at 24–48 hr, which then dropped to approximately 13%ID/g at 5 days. No accumulation of the ^{111}In was observed in the bone (Fig. 6A,C,E) over the period of study (1–7 days). Approximately 2.5%ID/g of bone was found at 24 hr in mice injected with B72.3 conjugated to all three chelates; this level dropped to approximately 1%ID/g at 7 days (Fig. 6A,C,E).

Significant differences were observed in the biodistribution of the ^{88}Y-labeled B72.3 IgG modified by the SCN-Bz-EDTA, CA-DTPA, and SCN-Bz-DTPA chelate conjugates. The yttrium coupled to B72.3 using the SCN–Bz–

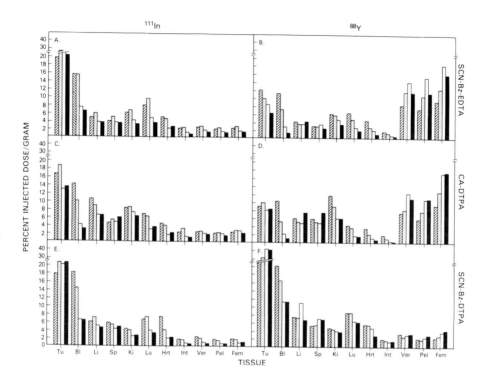

Figure 6 Biodistribution of B72.3 IgG labeled with ^{111}In or ^{88}Y in tumor-bearing mice. Athymic mice bearing LS-174T, human colon carcinoma xenografts, were injected i.v. with approximately 2.5 μCi of ^{111}In-labeled (A, C, and E) or 0.5 μCi of ^{88}Y-labeled (B, D, and F) B72.3 IgG. The MAb was modified with either SCN-Bz-EDTA (A and B), CA-DTPA (C and D), or SCN-Bz-DTPA (E and F) chelate conjugates. Mice (four per group) were sacrificed at 24 hr (▨), 48 hr (▨), 120 (▫), or 168 hr (■) the percentage of the injected dose per gram was determined. The standard error of the mean was less than 4% of the average values for most of the tissues. Tu, tumor; Bl, blood; Li, liver; Sp, spleen; Ki, kidneys; Lu, lungs; Hrt, heart; Int, intestines; Ver, vertebrae; Pel, pelvis; Fem, femur. (From Roselli et al. [34].)

EDTA or CA-DTPA chelate conjugates cleared the blood rapidly, with only approximately 1.2%ID/g remaining at 7 days postinjection (Fig. 6B,D). The ^{88}Y-SCN-Bz-DTPA-B72.3 showed a slower blood clearance, with 11%ID/g remaining in the blood at 7 days (Fig. 6F). The accumulation of yttrium in the tumor exhibited an inverse correlation with the blood clearance. The mice injected with the SCN-Bz-DTPA–conjugated B72.3 had higher levels of ^{88}Y in the tumors, with approximately 40%ID/g at 5–7 days postinjection of the MAb, in contrast to only 6–8%ID/g in the tumor of the mice injected with the SCN-Bz-EDTA or CA-DTPA–conjugated B72.3.

The most important differences among the three chelates coupled to the B72.3 IgG were in the radionuclide uptake in the bone. The level of the ^{88}Y rose as a function of time in the bones of the mice injected with the SCN-Bz-EDTA– and CA-DTPA–conjugated IgG from approximately 8 and 7%ID/g at 24 hr to over 14 and 11%ID/g, respectively, in both the vertebrae and the pelvis at 5 days postinjection of the labeled MAbs. Slightly higher levels were observed in the femurs of all groups of mice. Mice injected with the ^{88}Y-SCN-Bz-DTPA-B72.3 showed considerably lower levels of yttrium in the bone, with only 3%ID/g at 5 days postinjection.

Studies were undertaken to determine whether the radioactivity found in the bone was localized in the bone marrow or in the cortical bone. The bone marrow was removed from the femurs by extensive washing. At 24 hr postinjection of ^{88}Y-B72.3 IgG modified by the SCN-Bz-EDTA and CA-DTPA chelate conjugates, over 90% of the radioactivity was associated with the cortical bone. The percentage of the ^{88}Y in the cortical bone increased as a function of time; 97% of the total bone radioactivity was found in the cortical bone at 7 days. The majority of the radioactivity in the bone of mice injected with ^{88}Y-labeled B72.3 modified by the SCN-Bz-DTPA chelate conjugate, however, was associated with the bone marrow at 24 hr post-injection of the MAb. As the ^{88}Y-SCN-Bz-DTPA–conjugated MAb cleared the blood pool, the activity in the bone marrow decreased; therefore, the percentage of the remaining activity found in the cortical bone increased with time to approximately 80% at 7 days. The total activity in the bone for the ^{88}Y-SCN-Bz-DTPA-B72.3 was only 3.6%ID/g at 7 days.

The difference between yttrium and indium biodistribution after administration of labeled MAbs illustrates the difficulties in using ^{111}In-labeled MAbs to predict the biodistribution and dosimetry of ^{90}Y-labeled MAbs. Although a given chelate conjugate may give a favorable biodistribution with ^{111}In, the biodistribution of yttrium in that chelate conjugate may be very different. Through the use of an appropriate chelate, such as SCN-Bz-DTPA, for attaching yttrium and indium to the MAb, one can minimize loss of the radiometal from the chelate and obtain similar biodistributions using both indium and yttrium. The low levels of bone uptake of the ^{88}Y-SCN-Bz-DTPA-B72.3 is especially important in minimizing marrow toxicity. The high tumor-to-bone ratios obtained with SCN-Bz-DTPA suggest the potential utility of ^{90}Y for radioimmunotherapy using this type of chelate conjugate.

ANALYSIS OF RECOMBINANT/CHIMERIC FORMS OF B72.3

In our studies, more than 60% of the patients who received B72.3 have developed an immunological response to murine IgG after a single injection [35,36]. In an attempt to minimize the immune response of these patients to the administered murine MAb, a recombinant form of the murine B72.3 and then a recombinant/chimeric antibody were developed, using the variable regions of the murine B72.3 and human heavy-chain (γ 4) and light-chain (k) constant regions [36,37]. Both the recombinant B72.3 (rB72.3) and the recombinant/chimeric B72.3 [cB72.3(γ_4)] IgGs maintain the tissue binding and idiotypic specificity of the native murine IgG [38]. The native B72.3 (nB72.3), rB72.3, and cB72.3(γ_4) IgGs were radiolabeled, and the biodistribution of these IgGs was studied in athymic mice bearing human colon carcinoma xenografts (LS-174T). Differences were observed between the cB72.3(γ_4) and the nB72.3 in the %ID/g that localized in the tumor. It was found that the whole-body clearance of the ^{125}I-cB72.3(γ_4) was consistently more rapid than that of ^{131}I-nB72.3. Only approximately 28%ID remained in the body at 48 hr postinjection of the cB72.3(γ_4) IgG versus approximately 68%ID of the nB72.3 IgG. This correlated with a more rapid blood clearance found with the cB72.3(γ_4) (see below). The somewhat lower absolute amount of the cB72.3(γ_4) in the tumor are mostly likely due to the observed more rapid clearance from the blood and body of the mouse compared to the nB72.3 and rB72.3. All three forms [nB72.3, rB72.3, and cB72.3(γ_4)] of the IgG, however, were able to localize to the colon tumor with similar RIs [38].

A recombinant/chimeric B72.3 with a human(γ_1) constant region has also been developed [39]. This cB72.3(γ_1) was characterized and shown to retain binding to TAG-72 and idiotypic properties similar to that of the nB72.3. Dual-label studies of coinjected cB72.3(γ_1) and nB72.3 revealed that both MAbs could efficiently localize to human tumor xenografts in athymic mice. Pharmacokinetic studies, analyzing the blood clearance of cB72.3(γ_1), cB72.3(γ_4), and nB72.3 in mice, showed that the nB72.3 ß-phase of clearance was slower than that of the other MAb forms (Fig. 7A). However, when the pharmacokinetic patterns of these three MAb forms were analyzed in monkeys, the cB72.3(γ_1) and the nB72.3 showed similar clearance curves, while the cB72.3(γ_4) showed a much slower plasma clearance (Fig 7B). One consideration for the construction of a cB72.3(γ_1) is that it may be active in mediating antibody-dependent cell-mediated cytotoxicity (ADCC), which has been previously demonstrated in vitro and in vivo with chimeric 17-1A constructs [40,41]. ADCC experiments using lymphokine-activated killer effector cells indicated better cell killing by the cB72.3(γ_1) than the nB72.3 [39,42].

The high degree of selective binding of MAb B72.3 to a wide range of carcinoma tissues, the preclinical studies (both diagnostic and therapeutic),

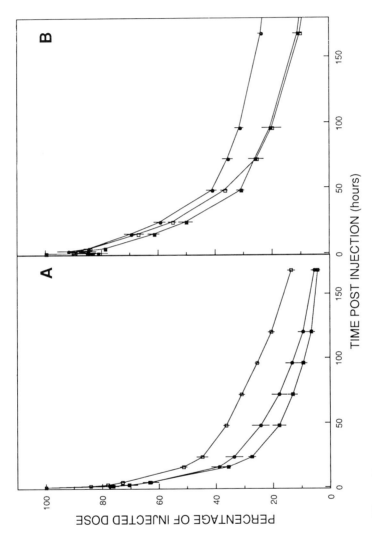

Figure 7 Clearance of radiolabeled native B72.3 (nB72.3) and chimeric B72.3 (cB72.3) MAbs from the plasma of mice (A) and cynomolgus monkeys (B); cB72.3(γ_1) (■), cB72.3(γ_4) (●), and nB72.3 (□). (From Hutzell et al. [39].)

and recent clinical trials have all demonstrated the potential utility of MAb B72.3. Thus, MAb B72.3, as well as the second-generation MAbs against TAG-72 and the recombinant/chimeric forms of these MAbs, are viable candidates in various aspects of the management of cancer.

REFERENCES

1. Colcher D, Horan Hand P, Nuti M, Schlom J. A spectrum of monoclonal antibodies reactive with human mammary tumor cells. Proc Natl Acad Sci USA 1981; 78:3199–3203.
2. Stramignoni D, Bowen R, Atkinson BF, Schlom J. Differential reactivity of monoclonal antibodies with human colon adenocarcinomas and adenomas. Int J Cancer 1983; 31:543–52.
3. Thor A, Gorstein F, Ohuchi N, Szpak CA, Johnston WW, Schlom J. Tumor-associated glycoprotein (TAG-72) in ovarian carcinomas defined by monoclonal antibody B72.3. J Natl Cancer Inst 1986; 76:995–1006.
4. Thor A, Ohuchi N, Szpak CA, Johnston WW, Schlom J. Distribution of oncofetal antigen TAG-72 defined by monoclonal antibody B72.3. Cancer Res 1986; 46:3118–24.
5. Nuti M, Teramoto YA, Mariani-Constantini R, Horan Hand P, Colcher D, Schlom J. A monoclonal antibody (B72.3) defines patterns of distribution of a novel tumor-associated antigen in human mammary carcinoma cell populations. Int J Cancer 1982; 29:539–45.
6. Wolf BC, D'Emilia JC, Salem RR, DeCoste D, Sears HF, Gottlieb LS, Steele GD Jr. Detection of tumor-associated glycoprotein antigen (TAG-72) in premalignant lesions of the colon. J Natl Cancer Inst 1989; 81:1913–17.
7. Thor A, Viglione MJ, Muraro R, Ohuchi N, Schlom J, Gorstein F. Monoclonal antibody B72.3 reactivity with human endometrium: a study of normal and malignant tissues. Int J Gynecol Pathol 1987; 6:235–47.
8. Horan Hand P, Nuti M, Colcher D, Schlom J. Definition of antigenic heterogeneity and modulation among human mammary carcinoma cell populations using monoclonal antibodies to tumor-associated antigens. Cancer Res 1983; 43:728–35.
9. Friedman E, Thor A, Horan Hand P, Schlom J. Surface expression of tumor-associated antigens in primary cultured human colonic epithelial cells from carcinomas, benign tumors, and normal tissues. Cancer Res 1988; 45:5648–55.
10. Horan Hand P, Colcher D, Salomon D, Ridge J, Noguchi P, Schlom J. Influence of spatial configuration of carcinoma cell populations on the expression of a tumor-associated glycoprotein. Cancer Res 1985; 45:833–40.
11. Greiner JW, Horan Hand P, Noguchi P, Fisher P, Pestka S, Schlom J. Enhanced expression of surface tumor associated antigens on human breast and colon tumor cells after recombinant leukocyte α -interferon treatment. Cancer Res 1984; 44:3208–14.

12. Greiner JW, Tobi M, Fisher PB, Langer JA, Pestka S. Differential responsiveness of cloned mammary carcinoma cell populations to the human recombinant leukocyte interferon enhancement of tumor antigen expression. Int J Cancer 1985; 36:159–66.

13. Kantor J, Tran R, Greiner J, Pestka S, Fisher PB, Shively JE, Schlom J. Modulation of carcinoembryonic antigen messenger RNA levels in human colon carcinoma cells by recombinant human γ-interferon. Cancer Res 1989; 49:2651–5.

14. Guadagni F, Schlom J, Johnston WW, Szpak CA, Goldstein D, Smalley R, Simpson JF, Borden EC, Pestka S, Greiner JW. Selective interferon-induced enhancement of tumor-associated antigens on a spectrum of freshly isolated human adenocarcinoma cells. J Natl Cancer Inst 1989; 81:502–12.

15. Johnson VG, Schlom J, Paterson AJ, Bennett J, Magnani JL, Colcher D. Analysis of a human tumor-associated glycoprotein (TAG-72) identified by monoclonal antibody B72.3. Cancer Res 1986; 46:850–7.

16. Paterson AJ, Schlom J, Sears HF, Bennett J, Colcher D. A radioimmunoassay for the detection of a tumor-associated glycoprotein (TAG-72) using monoclonal antibody B72.3. Int J cancer 1986; 37:659–66.

17. Muraro R, Kuroki M, Wunderlich D, Poole DJ, Colcher D, Thor A, Greiner JW, Simpson JF, Molinolo A, Noguchi P, Schlom J. Generation and characterization of B72.3 second generation monoclonal antibodies reactive with the tumor associated glycoprotein 72 antigen. Cancer Res 1988; 48:4588–96.

18. Sheer DG, Schlom J, Cooper HL. Purification and composition of the human tumor-associated glycoprotein (TAG-72) defined by monoclonal antibodies CC49 and B72.3. Cancer Res 1988; 48:6811–8.

19. Katari RS, Fernsten PD, Schlom J. Characterization of the shed form of the human tumor-associated glycoprotein (TAG-72) from serous effusions of patients with different types of carcinomas. Cancer Res 1990; 50:4885–90.

20. Klug TL, Sattler MA, Colcher D, Schlom J. Monoclonal antibody immunoradiometric assay for an antigenic determinant (CA 72) on a novel pancarcinoma antigen (TAG-72). Int J Cancer 1986; 38:661–9.

21. Gero EJ, Colcher D, Ferroni P, Melsheimer R, Giani S, Schlom J, Kaplan P. The CA 72-4 radioimmunoassay for the detection of the TAG-72 carcinoma associated antigen in serum of patients. J Clin Lab Analysis 1989; 3:360–9.

22. Ohuchi N, Gero E, Mori S, Akimoto M, Matoba N, Nishihira T, Hirayama K, Colcher D, Schlom J. Clinical evaluation of CA 72-4 immunoradiometric assay for serum TAG-72 in patients with carcinoma. J Tumor Marker Oncol 1990; 5:1–10.

23. Ohuchi N, Mori S, Gero E, Colcher D, Mochizuki F, Nishihira T, Akimoto M, Hirayama K, Matoba N, Kaplan PM, Schlom J. Serum levels of tumor-associated glycoprotein (TAG-72) in patients with carcinoma detected by CA 72-4 radioimmunometric assay (submitted for publication).

24. Colcher D, Keenan AM, Larson SM, Schlom J. Prolonged binding of a radiolabeled monoclonal antibody (B72.3) used for the in situ radioimmunodetection of human colon carcinoma xenografts. Cancer Res 1984; 44:5744–51.

25. Esteban JM, Schlom J, Mornex F, Colcher D. Radioimmunotherapy of athymic mice bearing human colon carcinomas with monoclonal antibody B72.3: histologic

and autoradiographic study of effects on tumors and normal organs. Eur J Cancer Clin Oncology 1987; 23:643–55.

26. Schlom J, Molinolo A, Simpson JF, Siler K, Roselli M, Hinkle G, Houchens DP, Colcher D. Advantage of dose fractionation in monoclonal antibody-targeted radioimmunotherapy. J Natl Cancer Inst 1990; 82:763–71.

27. Wessels BW, Rogus RD. Radionuclide selection and model absorbed dose calculation for radiolabeled tumor associated antibodies. Med Phys 1984; 11:638–45.

28. O'Brien HA Jr. Overview of radionuclides useful for radioimmunoimaging/radioimmunotherapy and current status of preparing radiolabeled antibodies. In: (Burchiel SW, Rhodes BA, eds.) Radioimmunoimaging and radioimmunotherapy. New York: Elsevier 1983:161–9.

29. DeNardo SJ, Jungerman JA, DeNardo GL, Lagunas-Solar MC, Cole WC, Meares CF. The choice of radionuclides for radioimmunotherapy. In: (Thiessen JW, Paras P, eds) The developing role of short-lived radionuclides in nuclear medicine practice. 1982, DOE Symposium Series, Washington, DC, May 3-5, 1982; Office of Scientific and Technical Information, U.S. Department of Energy, Oak Ridge, TN.

30. Hnatowich DJ, Layne WW, Childs RL. The preparation and labeling of DTPA-coupled albumin. Int J Appl Radiat Isotopes 1982; 33:327–32.

31. Krejcarek GE, Tucker KL. Covalent attachment of chelating groups to macromolecules. Biochem Biophys Res Commun 1977; 77:581–5.

32. Meares CF, McCall MJ, Reardan DT, Goodwin DA, Diamanti CI, McTigue M. Conjugation of antibodies with bifunctional chelating agents: Isothiocyanate and bromoacetamide reagents, methods of analysis, and subsequent addition of metal ions. Anal Biochem 1984; 142:68–78.

33. Brechbiel MW, Gansow OA, Atcher RW, Schlom J, Esteban J, Simpson D, Colcher D. Synthesis of I-(*p*-isothiocyanatobenzyl) derivatives of DTPA and EDTA. Antibody labeling and tumor imaging studies. Inorgan Chem 1986; 25:2772–81.

34. Roselli M, Schlom J, Gansow OA, Raubitschek A, Mirzadeh S, Brechbiel MW, Colcher D. Comparative biodistributions of yttrium and indium labeled monoclonal antibody B72.3 in athymic mice bearing human colon carcinoma xenografts. J Nucl Med 1989; 30:672–82.

35. Colcher D, Milenic DE, Ferroni P, Carrasquillo JA, Reynolds JC, Roselli M, Larson SM, Schlom J. In vivo fate of monoclonal antibody B72.3 in patients with colorectal cancer. J Nucl Med 1990; 31:1133–42.

36. Reynolds JC, Del Vecchio S, Sakahara H, Lora ME, Carrasquillo JA, Neumann, RD, Larson SM. Anti-murine antibody response to mouse monoclonal antibodies: clinical findings and implications. Nucl Med Biol 1989; 16:121–5.

37. Whittle N, Adair J, Lloyd C, Jenkins L, Devine J, Schlom J, Raubitschek A, Colcher D, Bodmer M. Expression in COS cells of a mouse-human chimaeric B72.3 antibody. Protein Engin 1987; 1:499–505.

38. Colcher D, Milenic D, Roselli M, Raubitschek A, Yarranton G, King D, Adair J, Whittle N, Bodmer M, Schlom J. Characterization and biodistribution of recombinant and recombinant/chimeric constructs of monoclonal antibody B72.3. Cancer Res 1989; 49:1738–45.

39. Hutzell P, Kashmiri S, Colcher D, Primus J, Horan Hand P, Roselli M, Finch M, Yarranton G, Bodmer M, Whittle N, King D, Loullis CC, McCoy, DW, Callahan R, Schlom J. Generation and characterization of a recombinant/chimeric B72.3 (human γ_1) Cancer Res 1991; 51:181–9.

40. Steplewski Z, Sun LK, Shearman CW, Ghrayeb J, Dadonna P, Koprowski H. Biological activity of human-mouse IgG1, IgG2, IgG3, and IgG4 chimeric monoclonal antibodies with antitumor specificity. Proc Natl Acad Sci USA 1988; 85:4852–6.

41. Shaw DR, Khazaeli MB, LoBuglio AF. Mouse/human chimeric antibodies to a tumor-associated antigen: biologic activity of the four human IgG subclasses. J Natl Cancer Inst 1988; 80:1553–9.

42. Primus FJ, Pendurthi TK, Hutzell P, Kashmiri S, Callahan R, Schlom J. Chimeric B72.3 mouse-human (γ_1) antibody directs the lysis of tumor cells by lymphokine-activated killer cells. Cancer Immunol Immunother 1990; 31:349–59.

43. Ohuchi N, Thor A, Nose M, Fujita J, Kyogoku M, Schlom J. Tumor-associated glycoprotein (TAG-72) detected in adenocarcinomas and benign lesions of the stomach. Int J Cancer 1986; 38:643–50.

44. Takasaki H, Tempero MA, Uchida E, Buchler M, Ness MJ, Burnett DA, Metzgar RS, Colcher D, Schlom J, Pour PM. Comparative studies on the expression of tumor-associated glycoprotein (TAG-72), CA 19-9 and DU-PAN-2 in normal, benign and malignant pancreatic tissue. Int J Cancer 1988; 42:681–6.

3

Imaging of Colorectal Carcinoma with ^{131}I B72.3 Monoclonal Antibody

Jorge A. Carrasquillo

National Cancer Institute, National Institutes of Health, Bethesda, Maryland

INTRODUCTION

Multiple studies on imaging colorectal carcinoma with a variety of radiolabeled polyclonal and monoclonal antibodies (MAbs) have appeared in the literature [1-7]. Several tumor-associated antigens have been identified as targets for radioimmunoscintigraphy (for review, see Ref. 8). These include carcino-9 embryonic antigen (CEA) and other antigens targeted by MAbs 17-1A, 19-9, 791T/36, and B72.3 (anti-TAG-72). The National Institutes of Health (NIH) group has reported on the imaging of patients with colorectal carcinoma targeting TAG-72 tumor–associated antigen with ^{131}I B72.3 MAb [9-12]. These studies included pharmacokinetic analyses as well as surgical and pathological correlations. These preliminary findings laid the groundwork for subsequent studies examining the effects of a variety of radiolabeling strategies and alternate routes of administration. In this chapter, we will review the studies carried out at NIH that utilized the intravenous administration of ^{131}I B72.3 in patients with colorectal carcinoma.

The content of this chapter does not necessarily reflect the views or policies of the Department of Health and Human Services, nor does mention of trade names, commercial products, or organizations imply endorsements by the U.S. Government.

ANTIGEN AND ANTIBODY

TAG-72 is a high-molecular-weight, mucin-like, tumor-associated antigen [13]. It is present in several epithelial-derived carcinomas [14–16], including approximately 85% of colorectal carcinomas, and therefore it is considered pancarcinoma. Because it is also present in some fetal tissues, TAG-72 is considered an oncofetal antigen [17]. Cross-reactivity with some normal adult tissues has been reported, including binding to normal secretory endometrium and some benign neoplasias and normal colon tissues from patients with colorectal carcinoma [18]. Nevertheless, this cross-reactivity has not had an adverse impact on imaging studies.

B72.3 is a murine IgG1 MAb, produced by immunizing Balb/c mice with a membrane-rich fraction from a human carcinoma metastasis [19]. This antibody recognizes TAG-72. The antibodies used in our studies were purified from mouse ascites by ammonium sulfate precipitation and ion-exchange chromatography [20]. The purified IgG was tested according to the U.S. Food and Drug Administration (FDA) guidelines [21].

B72.3 was labeled with ^{131}I using the Iodogen method [22] and purified by gel filtration chromatography. The specific activity of the clinical preparations varied from 0.3 to 12.6 mCi/mg, and patients received from 0.8 to 10 mCi of ^{131}I. The quality control procedures showed a mean of 98% protein bound ^{131}I, and more than 80% of the ^{131}I B72.3 remained immunoreactive, based on sequential solid-phase radioimmunoassays (RIAs) [20].

STUDY DESIGN

The goals of the study included evaluation of pharmacokinetics, dose dependency, specificity of tumor binding, and imaging ability of ^{131}I B72.3. Thirty-five patients who were followed by the surgery branch of the National Cancer Institute (NCI) and who had histologically confirmed colorectal carcinoma were studied [11]. The protocol was approved by the Institutional Human Research Committee of the NCI and all patients gave their informed consent. The group consisted of 22 men and 13 women, with a mean age of 51 years (range 16–70 years). Two patients had primary colon tumors (in one patient this was the second primary) and the others had metastatic colon carcinoma. Thirty-two patients had surgical exploration following antibody infusion in an attempt to debulk or cure them of their tumor. Thirty patients had evidence of metastatic disease by conventional radiographic workup. A rising CEA was the only sign of recurrence in three patients, and two patients had primary tumors detected by colonoscopy.

IMAGING RESULTS

The effect of protein mass on tumor localization was evaluated by using doses of 0.16–20 mg of MAb and 0.8–10 mCi of ^{131}I. The antibody was administered intravenously as a 1-hr. infusion. The patients were imaged within 2 hrs. of infusion and daily thereafter until the day prior to surgery (range 4–15 days, mean 8 days). Anterior and posterior whole-body images as well as multiple spot views (5–10 min) were obtained using an extra large field-of-view gamma camera. The images were interpreted as positive when focal areas of increased uptake were seen in the analog images in regions not corresponding to sites of physiological uptake (blood pool, bladder, and thyroid). The scan results were correlated with radiographic and surgical findings.

Sixteen of thirty-five patients had positive scans. The anatomic distribution of lesions represented the usual metastatic sites of colon cancer. Table 1 indicates the sites of tumor involvement and the imaging results for each site. No difference in tumor detection ability was observed at the different dose levels of B72.3 (Table 2). Scans accurately identified tumor lesions in the liver, bone, orbit, rectum, colon, cecum, pelvis, and diffusely in the peritoneal cavity. By scan, the smallest lesion detected was 2.5 cm in diameter, with most detected lesions being 4 cm or larger.

Gamma camera images showed that the radiolabeled antibody distributed predominantly in the blood pool, with very little selective accumulation in normal organs (Fig. 1). However, in four patients with circulating antigen and evidence of immune complexes as determined by high-performance liquid chromatographic (HPLC) serum assay, there was mildly increased splenic activity with no tumor detected at this site.

The optimum time for imaging was found to be about 1 week post-administration when the background activity had decreased and tumor-to-nontumor ratios were greatest. Several hepatic metastases presented as cold lesions on early images; these lesions demonstrated equal or greater intensity than the normal liver tissue at the delayed imaging times (Fig. 2), indicating a slower access to tumor and more prolonged retention in liver metastases than in normal liver.

PHARMACOKINETICS

Plasma clearance was determined by gamma-counting serial post-infusion plasma samples obtained up to the time of surgery. The MAb circulated in the blood pool with a mean terminal half-life of 65 hr. (range 32–106 hr.), which was not significantly different between dose levels. Whole-body retention of ^{131}I was determined by probe counts. The whole-body radioactivity cleared with a mean half-life of 82 hrs. Escalating doses of ^{131}I B72.3 (up to 20 mg) had

Table 1 Scan Results by Site of Involvement

| | Primary tumors | Metastatic tumors | | | | |
		Peritoneum	Liver	Lung	Bone	Retroperitoneum	Spleen
Positive	1	6	9	0	1	0	0
Total	2	15	17	6	1	5	1

Source: Data from Ref. 11.

Table 2 Scan Results by Dose[a]

Dose[b]	0.28 mg	1.06 mg	4.18mg	19.2 mg
Positive	6	7	1	2
Total	11	16	3	5

[a]Data from reference 11.
[b]Mean mg dose of B72.3 administered.
Source: Data from Ref. 11.

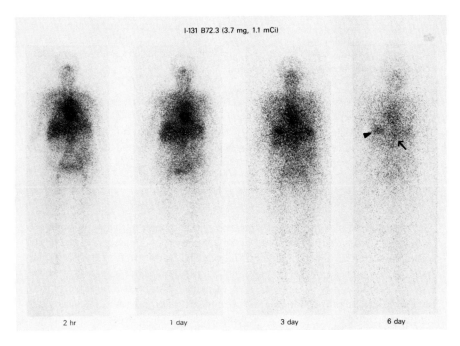

Figure 1   Serial anterior whole-body images from patient with metastatic adenocarcinoma of the colon to the liver. The scans were obtained after i.v. injection of 1.1 mCi, 3.7 mg of ¹³¹I B72.3. There is a slow clearance of radioactivity from the blood pool and whole body. At 2 hr and at 1 day, there is a normal-appearing liver, but at 3 and 6 days, when the blood pool and liver background have decreased, there is evidence of metastatic disease to the right lobe of the liver (arrowhead). A second metastasis to the left lobe of the liver (arrow) is not clearly seen because of the high adjacent background in the heart and left upper quadrant. (Data from Ref. 11.)

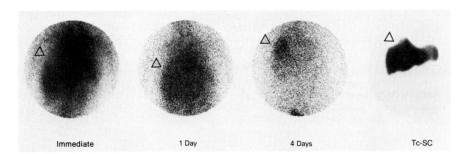

| Immediate | 1 Day | 4 Days | Tc-SC |

Figure 2   Serial anterior views of the chest (2 mCi, 0.34 mg of [131]I B72.3) demonstrating a photopenic region in the liver (arrowhead) corresponding to a large colon cancer metastasis. At 1 day postinfusion the lesion has equal activity to the normal liver, while at 4 days the lesion has more uptake than the surrounding normal liver and background. A ^{99m}Tc sulfur colloid scan (Tc-SC) shows a large metastasis. (Data from Ref. 11.)

no effect on the plasma or whole-body clearances (Table 3). Nineteen of thirty-four patients evaluated had elevated levels of TAG-72, but this did not appear to affect clearance from the plasma or the whole body or to prevent tumor imaging. There was a good correlation between elevated TAG-72 antigen levels and tumor imaging [11].

TISSUE CORRELATION

The biopsy data were analyzed from the initial 20 patients injected with [131]I B72.3 and subsequently evaluated by laparotomy [9]. All surgical specimens were labeled according to organ and anatomical location, and a representative specimen of each was immediately weighed and counted in a gamma counter to establish the activity (cpm) per gram of tissue. These specimens were then fixed in formalin, embedded in paraffin, and sectioned for routine histological studies and immunohistological determinations. The percentage of tumor present in each section was determined by light microscopy. Representative nontumor tissues (usually liver, margin of resection of colon, and/or small intestines) were selected, and their activities in counts per gram were averaged. A radiolocalization index (RI) value was defined as the ratio of the uptake of ^{131}I-labeled MAb per gram of histologically confirmed tumor (>20% tumor cells) to that per gram of histologically confirmed normal tissue. The average values (cpm/g) from biopsy of normal liver and/or intestinal tissue of each patient were normalized to 1.0. RIs > 3.0 were arbitrarily considered as "positive" for these studies. As can be seen in Table 4, at least one tumor lesion in 17 of 20 patients had an RI > 3.0. In eight of the patients, all 50 tumor lesions biopsied had RIs > 3.0 (Table 4). Five of the patients displayed 26 lesions with RIs > 10.0 (Table 4). In total, 99 of 142 (70%) carcinoma lesions displayed RIs > 3.0. There was no effect of IgG dose, ^{131}I activity (mCi), or specific activity on the RI observed in the 20 patients.

A total of 198 of 210 histologically confirmed normal tissues biopsied showed a negative RI (≤3.0). In 12 patients, all apparently normal tissues biopsied had negative RIs. Twelve normal biopsy specimens from eight patients showed RIs > 3.0. In all but two cases, high RIs were seen in spleen biopsies. It is possible that this was due to the presence of immune complexes in spleen.

The percentage of injected dose of ^{131}I-labeled MAb B72.3 per gram of carcinoma tissue at the time of surgery (approximately 6–7 days postadministration) ranged from 0.0002 to 0.01 for the patients studied.

An ^{125}I-labeled isotype-matched MAb (BL-3) was used as a control in four patients to delineate the selective binding of MAb B72.3 for colon carcinoma lesions. MAb BL-3 is a murine IgG1 antiidiotype MAb that is reactive with a B-cell lymphoma [9]. Similar amounts (1.5 mg) of ^{125}I-labeled BL-3 and ^{131}I-labeled B72.3 were coinjected into each patient. While tumor tissues had 2–4 times more binding with B72.3 than with BL-3, equivalent amounts of both BL-3 and B72.3 were observed in histologically normal tissues, such as colon, small intestine, liver, peritoneum, omentum, lymph nodes, and gallbladder.

TOXICITY

The intravenous infusions of B72.3 were well tolerated with no side effects. Fifty-two percent of the patients developed human antimouse antibodies (HAMA) [23]. The development of HAMA did not result in any side effects. No repeat injections were given to any of the patients studied; therefore, the effect of HAMA on biodistribution was not assessed.

DISCUSSION

We have documented the specificity of tumor targeting by ^{131}I B72.3 in colorectal cancer. In contrast to other studies, very little cross-reactivity with normal tissues was observed and there was no evidence of a MAb dose effect on pharmacokinetics or tumor imaging. Because of its limited sensitivity of tumor imaging (16 of 35 patients), ^{131}I B72.3 is unlikely to be useful clinically. Nevertheless, our results showing selective tumor uptake in 70% of the tumors biopsied warrant further studies evaluating strategies that may improve tumor uptake. These approaches include up-regulating antigen expression with interferon, using other radiolabeling methods, using alternate routes of administration, and using chimeric antibodies or a second generation of antibodies directed at the same antigen but of higher affinity.

Table 3 Dose Effect of B72.3 on Whole-Body and Plasma Retention

Dose (mean ± SD) B72.3	0.28 ± 0.09 mg (n = 11)	1.04 ± 0.2 mg (n = 16)	4.18 ± 0.71 mg (n = 3)	19.2 ± 0.8 mg (n = 5)
Whole-body retention[a]				
0 day[b]	100	100	100	100
1 day	79	78	83	80
2 days	61	60	69	66
3 days	51	58	61	50
Plasma retention[a]				
0 hr[b]	95	92	88	82
1 hr	91	90	89	75
2 hr	78	80	80	75
1 day	62	57	55	63
2 days	41	41	40	42
3 days	37	30	30	32
6 days	9	12	15	13

[a]Mean percent of the injected dose retained in the whole body or plasma.
[b] 0 = end of the 1-hr antibody infusion.
Source: Data from Ref. 11.

Table 4 Radiolocalization Indices of Tumor and Normal Tissue Biopsies of Patients Given Injections of ^{131}I-Labeled B72.3 IgG

Patient	Tumor RIs		Tumor lesions[a] (RI)			Normal tissues[b] (RI)		
	Minimum	Maximum	≤3	3-10	>10	≤3	3-10	>10
J.P.	8.5	29.6	0[c]	2	2	6	0	2
M.P.	5.3	45.8	0	5	13	8	0	0
H.B.	5.1	32.6	0	9	4	4	0	2
H.K.	10.3	10.3	0	0	1	20	0	0
P.H.	2.4	17.3	2	18	6	5	0	0
M.L.	4.8	8.9	0	3	0	20	1	0
B.B.	4.4	7.4	0	5	0	4	0	0
D.F.	3.9	7.3	0	5	0	16	1	0
C.C.	5.5	5.5	0	1	0	13	0	0
E.S.	2.3	5.3	1	4	0	8	0	0
E.L.	2.9	4.1	1	1	0	6	0	0
H.L.	1.1	8.2	10	9	0	3	0	0
T.R.	2.1	4.2	1	2	0	10	1	0
M.S.	1.4	4.5	3	5	0	15	2	0
H.F.	2.2	4.0	1	1	0	15	0	0
R.C.	2.0	3.4	1	1	0	3	2	0
E.P.	0.8	5.3	13	2	0	5	0	0
C.M.	1.7	2.4	5	0	0	7	0	0
J.D.	1.3	2.4	4	0	0	19	1	0
J.R.	1.4	1.4	1	0	0	11	0	0

[a] The average RI value of all tumor lesions obtained for a given patient.
[b] Spleen ($n = 4$); lymph nodes ($n = 2$); peritoneum ($n = 2$); ileum ($n = 2$); omentum ($n = 1$); gallbladder ($n = 1$).
[c] Number of specimens with the indicated RI.

ACKNOWLEDGMENTS

The work presented here is the result of the collaborative efforts of the Laboratory of Tumor Immunology and Biology, the Radiation Oncology Branch, Surgery Branch, and the Laboratory of Pathology, of the NCI, and the Department of Nuclear Medicine, Warren G. Magnuson Clinical Center.

REFERENCES

1. Goldenberg DM, DeLand FH, Kim E, Bennett S, Primus FJ, Van Nagell JR, Estes N, DeSinome P, Rayburn P. Use of radiolabeled antibodies to carcinoembryonic antigen for the detection and localization of diverse cancers by external photoscanning. N Engl J Med 1978; 298:1384-6.
2. Mach J-P, Carrel S, Forni M, Ritschard J, Donath A, Alberto P. Tumor localization of radiolabeled antibodies against carcinoembryonic antigen in patients with carcinoma. N Engl J Med 1980; 303:5-10.
3. Mach J-P, Buchegger F, Forni M, Ritschard J, Berche C, Lumbroso JD, Schreyer M, Girardet C, Accolla RS, Carrell S. Use of radiolabeled monoclonal anti-CEA antibodies for the detection of human carcinomas by external photoscanning and tomoscintigraphy. Immunol Today 1981; 2:239-47.
4. Mach J-P, Chatal JF, Lumbroso JD, Buchegger F, Forni M, Ritschard J, Berche C, Douillard JY, Carrel S, Heryln M, Steplewski Z, Koprowski H. Tumor localization in patients by radiolabeled monoclonal antibodies against colon carcinoma. Cancer Res 1983; 43:5593-5600.
5. Chatal JF, Saccavini JC, Fumoleau P, Douillard JY, Curtet C, Kremer M, Le Maevel B, Koprowski H. Immunoscintigraphy of colon carcinoma. J Nucl Med 1984; 25:307-14.
6. Moldofsky PJ, Powe J, Mulhern CB, Hammond N, Sears HF, Gatenby RA, Steplewski Z, Koprowski H. Metastatic colon carcinoma detection with radiolabeled F(ab')2 monoclonal antibody fragments. Radiology 1983; 149:549-55.
7. Hnatowich DJ, Griffin TW, Kusciuczyk C, Rusckowski M, Childs RL, Mattis JA, Shealy D, Doherty PW. Pharmacokinetics of an indium-111-labeled monoclonal antibody in cancer patients. J Nucl MEd 1985; 26(8):849-58.
8. Carrasquillo JA. Radioimmunoscintigraphy with polyclonal or monoclonal antibodies. In: Zalutzky M, ed. Antibodies in radiodiagnosis and therapy. Boca Raton, FL:CRC Press, 1988: 169-98.
9. Colcher D, Esteban JM, Carrasquillo JA, Sugarbaker P, Reynolds JC, Bryant G, Larson SM, Schlom J. Quantitative analyses of selective radiolabeled monoclonal antibody localization in metastatic lesions of colorectal cancer patients. Cancer Res 1987; 47:1185-9.
10. Esteban JM, Colcher D, Sugarbaker D, Carrasquillo JA, Bryant G, Thor A, Reynolds JC, Larson SM, Schlom J. Quantitative and qualitative aspects of radiolocalization in colon cancer patients of intravenously administered MoAb B72.3. Int J Cancer 1987; 29:50.

11. Carrasquillo JA, Sugarbaker P, Colcher D, Reynolds JC, Esteban J, Bryant G, Keenan AN, Perentesis P, Yokoyama K, Simpson DE, Ferroni P, Farkas R, Schlom J, Larson SM. Radioimmunoscintigraphy of colon cancer with I-131 B72.3 monoclonal antibody. J Nucl Med 1988; 29:1022–30.

12. Yokoyama K, Carrasquillo JA, Chang AE, Colcher D, Roselli M, Sugarbaker P, Sindelar W, Reynolds JC, Perentesis P, Gansow OA, Francis B, Adams R, Finn R, Schlom J, Larson SM. Differences in biodistribution of In-111 and I-131-labeled B72.3 monoclonal antibodies in patients with colorectal cancer. J Nucl Med 1989; 30:320–7.

13. Johnson VG, Schlom J, Paterson AJ, Bennett J, Magnani JL, Colcher D. Analysis of a human tumor-associated glycoprotein (TAG-72) identified by monoclonal antibody B72.3. Cancer Res 1986; 46:850-7.

14. Stramignomi D, Bowen R, Atkinson BF, Schlom J. Differential reactivity of monoclonal antibodies with human colon adenocarcinomas and adenomas. Int J Cancer 1983; 31:543–52.

15. Nuti M, Teramoto YA, Mariani-Constatini R, Horan Hand P, Colcher D, Schlom J. A monoclonal antibody (B72.3) defines patterns of distribution of a novel tumor-associated antigen in human mammary carcinoma cell population. Int J Cancer 1982; 29:539–45.

16. Thor A, Gorstein F, Ohuchi N, Szpak CA, Johnston WW, Schlom J. Tumor-associated glycoprotein (TAG-72) in ovarian carcinomas defined by monoclonal antibody B72.3. J Natl Cancer Inst 1986; 76:995–1006.

17. Thor A, Ohuchi N, Szpak CA, Johnston WW, Schlom J. The distribution of oncofetal antigen TAG-72 recognized by monoclonal antibody B72.3. Cancer Res 1986; 46:3118–24.

18. Listrom MB, Little JV, McKinley M, Fenoglio-Preiser CM. Immunoreactivity of tumor-associated glycoprotein (TAG-72) in normal, hyperplastic, and neoplastic colon. Human Pathol 1989; 20(10):994–1000.

19. Colcher D, Hand P, Nuti M, Schlom J. A spectrum of monoclonal antibodies reactive with human mammary tumor cells. Proc Natl Acad Sci. USA 1981; 78:3199–3203.

20. Colcher D, Keenan AM, Larson SM, Schlom J. Prolonged binding of a radiolabeled monoclonal antibody (B72.3) used for onsite radioimmunodetection of human colon carcinoma xenografts. Cancer Res 1984; 44:5744–51.

21. Office of Biologics Research and Review Center for Drugs and Biologics, FDA. Points to consider in the manufacture of injectable monoclonal antibody products intended for human use in vivo. Available from the Dockets Management Branch, FDA, 5600 Fisher Lane, Rockville MD 20857.

22. Fraker PJ, Speck JC Jr. Protein and cell membrane iodinations with a sparingly soluble chloroamide, 1,3,4,6-techrachloro-3a, 6a-diphenylglycoluril. Biochem Biophys Res Commun 1978; 80:849–57.

23. Reynolds JC, Carrasquillo JA, Lora ME, et al. Measurements of human anti-murine antibodies in patients who received radiolabeled monoclonal antibodies. J Nucl Med 1987; 25:425–7.

4

Monoclonal Antibody B72.3 Immunoscintigraphy in the Follow-up of Patients with Colorectal Cancer

Secondo Lastoria and Marco Salvatore

University of Naples, 2nd Medical School and
National Cancer Institute "G. Pascale," Naples, Italy

INTRODUCTION

The prognosis of epithelial tumors is often negatively conditioned by a late diagnosis, and therapy is often ineffective because metastases have been developed. An early detection of recurrences and metastases is required during follow-up to address specific treatment.

The advent of hybridoma technology [1] has made large amounts of monoclonal antibodies (MAbs) available for clinical use. The challenge has been to utilize these biological tools as powerful agents in the diagnosis and therapy of human cancer [2,3]. Radiolabeled murine immunoglobulins reacting with colon cancer–associated antigens, such as carcinoembryonic antigen (CEA) [4–6] and non-CEA antigens, have frequently been investigated. Among these non-CEA antigens, the tumor-associated glycoprotein-72 (TAG-72) [7] has been widely studied. TAG-72 is a high-molecular-weight mucin-like glycoprotein (MW > 1,000,000), recognized by B72.3 MAb, a murine IgG1 that binds to 90% of colonic, gastric [8], and ovarian cancers [9], whereas it does not react with normal adult tissue with the exception of secretory endometrium [10].

Several studies of in vivo tumor targeting using radiolabeled B72.3 in patients with colorectal [11–13] and ovarian [14] cancer have already been published demonstrating the advantage of using this reagent to detect distant metastases and local recurrences. The rationale for this study was to verify the clinical role of radioimmunoscintigraphy (RIS) with labeled B72.3 in the workup of a large series of patients with colorectal cancer after surgery. In fact, in these patients the incidence of recurrences at anastomotic sites, involvement of locoregional lymph nodes, distant metastases, and peritoneal carcinomatosis is high. These localizations are usually underestimated using clinical examination, serum tumor marker assays, and currently available radiological techniques.

RIS with a suitable MAb, such as B72.3 IgG, might represent a noninvasive, sensitive, specific approach to solving diagnostic problems. The theoretical and practical advantages of RIS over other imaging procedures can be summarized in: (1) high specificity of tumor targeting, which is not affected by other causes (such as ultrasound reflection, paramagnetic properties, attenuation phenomena); (2) greater sensitivity than ultrasound and computed tomography in detecting peritoneal implants or abdominal metastases when ascites occurs; (3) ability to differentiate between recurrence and post-treatment fibrosis; and (4) utility as a unique baseline approach for subsequent immunotherapy based on the use of MAbs.

MATERIALS AND METHODS
Monoclonal Antibody and Labeling Procedure

B72.3 MAb has been generated using a membrane-enriched fraction of human mammary carcinoma metastasis to the liver [15]. B72.3 is a murine IgGl that shows reactivity for malignant and atypical lesions and can be considered a marker of malignant transformation [16].

One milligram of B72.3 was labeled with approximately 7–10 mCi of Na^{131}I, using the Iodogen method [17], in a glass vial precoated with Iodogen (250 μg). The labeling was carried out for 10 min at 22°C. Free ^{131}I was separated from the coupled MAb by anion-exchange chromatography Dowex 1X8 equilibrated with sterile phosphate buffer saline (PBS) with 3% human serum albumin. No aggregates were found in labeled preparations by high-performance liquid chromatography (HPLC) using TSK-G-3000-SW columns. Paper chromatography (methanol 85%) and paper electrophoresis (1 hr at 200 V, in PBS, pH 7.1) showed that more than 98% of ^{131}I was protein bound. The specific activities of injectable B72.3 ranged from 3 to 6 mCi/mg of protein.

Coupling of diethylenetriamine pentaacetic acid (DTPA) to B72.3 was performed using the bicyclic anhydride method [18]. One milligram of DTPA was incubated overnight at 4°C with whole B72.3 molecules previously dialyzed against NaHC°3 (pH 8.3). Uncoupled DTPA was separated from conjugated MAb by gel filtration on Sephadex G-50. Purified B72.3-DTPA was diluted to approximately 0.6 mg/ml with 0.01 M sodium bicarbonate (pH 7.8) containing 0.9% NaCl and 0.1% human serum albumin. Aliquots of 1 mg of B72.3-DTPA were buffered at pH 5.0 by adding 0.2 M sodium citrate buffer and labeled with 3–6 mCi of ^{111}In chloride. More than 98% of ^{111}In was protein-bound, as demonstrated by HPLC. The specific activity ranged from 2 to 3.5 mCi of ^{111}In per milligram of B72.3.

Evaluation of Labeled B72.3 Immunoreactivity

A commercially available direct binding assay using solid-phase antigen of colorectal tumors, (RhoCheck, Rhomed, Albuquerque, NM), was used to test the immunoreactivity of labeled B72.3 preparations before administration to the patients. Aliquots of labeled B72.3 (approximately 100,000 and 50,000 cpm/10 μl) were incubated with positive antigen extracts and a negative control antigen for 1 hr at 22°C. The samples were counted and successively washed twice with PBS. The supernatant of each washing was removed and the pellet was recounted to measure the percentage of radioactivity bound to the solid-phase antigen. Values ranging from 45 to 60% bound to the positive control were obtained for both ^{131}I and ^{111}In B72.3 preparations, the nonspecific binding of labeled B72.3 was <7%.

Patient Profiles

RIS was done in 68 patients (44 male and 24 female, age range 26–77 years) who had already undergone curative surgery. In nine patients with primary colon cancer, without distant metastases, RIS was performed before surgery. Fifty-nine patients were in follow-up from 6 to 36 months after surgery. The complete clinical workup included: computed tomography, ultrasound, chest x-ray, liver and spleen scanning, and serum marker assays (CEA and TAG–72). Thyroid block was obtained by oral administration of Lugol's solution, starting 2 days before the ^{131}I B72.3 injection and for the entire study.

Radioimmunoscintigraphy Protocol

One hour before the injection of the diagnostic dose, an intradermal skin test was performed in all patients using 0.1 ml of murine IgG (0.1 mg/ml) in phosphate buffer saline, with a saline control in the contralateral arm to evaluate the hypersensitivity to murine IgGs.

Hematopoietic, renal, and hepatic functions were tested before and 2 weeks after the injection of MAb. Labeled B72.3 was intravenously administered over a 2 min period. Serial blood samples were collected just before the injection and at 5, 10, 30 min, 1, 2, 4, 24 hr, and then daily up to 10 days after. Urine samples were collected daily for the entire study to determine the cumulative urinary excretion of radioactivity.

Imaging Technique

Planar images were obtained at 10 min. 2 hrs., and daily up to 7 days following the injection using a large-field-of-view gamma camera equipped with a high-energy collimator and connected with a dedicated computer. In some patients, to lower the background and optimize the detection of small lesions, the subtraction technique introduced by Granowska et al. [19] was used. Briefly, subtraction of early images (10 min. and 2 hrs.) from late images (72, 96 hrs.) was performed after correction for the physical decay of the isotope and careful replacement of the patient in the same positions during the entire study. This method eliminates some of the problems related to the use of isotopes with different energies. The exact replacement of the patient, to avoid movement artifacts, was ensured by radioactive sources placed on anatomical markers. Digital images were analyzed using the regions-of-interest technique to determine activity/time curves at tumor sites and for the whole body. Three different physicians reviewed the images to classify the study as positive or negative for B72.3 tumor targeting. Two of them did not know the results of the complete clinical workup.

Tissue Studies

Immunohistochemistry

The surgical specimens were snap-frozen in liquid nitrogen or fixed in 10% formalin and embedded in paraffin. The evaluation of TAG-72 expression was performed on cryostat 8 μm sections using the avidin-biotin complex (ABC) method [20]. The specificity of immunohistochemistry (IHC) was confirmed by the negative control obtained after omission and replacement of the specific MAb. The score of immunohistochemical findings was graded from 0 to 4+.

Ex Vivo Quantitative Autoradiography and Gamma Counting of Biopsies

In seven patients, the biopsies removed at surgery were classified, weighed, and counted in a gamma counter to measure the percentage of labeled B72.3 per gram of tumors and normal organs/tissues. Each specimen was frozen in liquid nitrogen and then sectioned for routine histological staining (hematoxylin/eosin, immunoperoxidase, and mucicarmin acid); 20 μm sections were used for ex vivo quantitative autoradiography (EV-QAR). The sections and 20 μm slices of known Na ^{131}I standards (range 0.1–30 μCi/g) were exposed to single-coated sensitive x-ray films for 7–10 days. The developed films were digitized by a computerized videocamera. The optical densities (ODs) of Na-^{131}I standards were plotted versus their specific activity (μCi/g), determined by gamma counting, to obtain a standard curve. The ODs measured in tissue sections were automatically converted to μCi/g. This approach has been used to determine both: (1) concentration of radioactivity/gram of tissue and (2) pattern of labeled B72.3 distribution within tumor sections with respect to their architecture.

RADIOIMMUNOSCINTIGRAPHIC STUDIES IN PATIENTS WITH COLON CANCER

No adverse reactions or toxicity has been observed after the skin test and the subsequent dose of labeled B72.3 in the 68 cases we investigated; whole blood cell count and hepatic and renal tests remained unchanged. Levels of human antimouse antibody (HAMA) were measurable in 14 of the 35 patients whose sera were tested before and 20 days after the first and unique i.v. administration of labeled B72.3 whole IgG.

In Vivo Pharmacokinetics of Labeled B72.3

[131]I-labeled B72.3 IgG plasma clearance was determined in 25 patients who received approximately 1 mg of protein. The first mean component had a half-life ($t^{1/2}$) ranging from 2 to 4.5 hr; the second component had a $t^{1/2}$ ranging from 60 to 85 hr. The average percent injected dose (ID) for each experimental time point that resulted in a better fit by a biexponential curve is shown in Figure 1. Levels of radioactivity greater than 95% were bound to the MAb through the entire study, as demonstrated by precipitation in trichloracetic acid. The radioactivity was measurable in the plasma, and no binding with circulating cells occurred.

The cumulative urinary excretion reached 15 ± 8% of ID at day 1 postinjection and 65 ± 22% at day 4; more than 98% of radioactivity collected in the urine was unbound iodine.

At 24 hr, uptake of labeled B72.3 was visualized in the liver, spleen, lung, and scrotum as well as in major vessels. In later images (from 32 to 144 hr) tumor sites were depicted, when tumor-B72.3 binding occurred, while background activity decreased.

Results in Human Studies

Primary Colorectal Cancer

For nine patients with primary tumor localized in the left colon ($n = 5$) and rectum ($n = 4$), the results of RIS with [131]I B72.3, endoscopy, and barium enema are summarized in Table 1. The tumor size ranged between 2 and 6 cm in diameter. Histologically, four tumors were classified as poorly and

PLASMA LEVELS OF ¹³¹I LABELED B72.3 MoAb

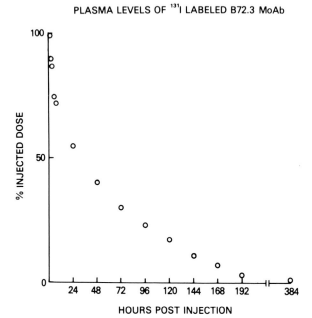

Figure 1 Plasma levels of ¹³¹I B72.3 determined in 25 patients reported as average for each time point. The blood clearance was followed up to 16 days after the i.v. injection. At 6 days 10% of injected dose was still circulating.

five as well-differentiated adenocarcinomas; by IHC six of eight tested biopsies showed TAG-72 expression, and in two a lack of antigen was demonstrated. In positive lesions, the expression of TAG-72 was highly heterogeneous. None of these patients had elevated levels of circulating TAG-72. Four colonic lesions were depicted by RIS; all the rectal lesions were missed. The identified tumors were 4 cm or greater in diameter.

The lack of detection for neoplastic nodules smaller than 4 cm when the antigen was expressed was basically due to the following causes: (1) expression of TAG-72 limited only to a few neoplastic clones (representing less than 20% of cellular component); (2) use of ¹³¹I, which has a gamma energy (364 Kev) that is too high for optimal image resolution (in addition, its beta emission with the long 8-day half-life limits the dose that can be safely injected); (3) high levels of circulating radioactivity during the first week after injection (10–28% of ID); and (4) nonuse of subtraction techniques or single-photon emission tomography to improve the tumor/background ratio and provide a better spatial resolution for relatively small lesions.

Table 1 Comparative Findings in Patients with Primary Colorectal Cancer Submitted to RIS with [131]I B72.3 MAb

No. of Cases	Dukes stage	RIS	Results of clinical workup		
			IHC	Endos.	B.E.
7	B	2/7	4/6[a]	7/7	7/7
2	C	2/2	2/2	2/2	2/2
Total		4/9	6/8	9/9	9/9

[a]One patient was operated on in a different institution and the IHC was not performed.
Endos., endoscopy; B.E., barium enema.

Metastatic Colorectal Cancer

In the group of 59 patients in follow-up, 41 had metastases, and 18 were disease-free according to the results of the complete clinical workup. Fifty-one patients received [131]I B72.3 (17 were disease free) and eight received ^{111}In-labeled-B72.3 MAb (1 was disease-free). At study entry, before antibody evaluation, 41 patients with active disease had 69 known lesions (Table 2) determined by computed tomography (CT), ultrasound (US), endoscopy, or clinical examination. After B72.3 imaging, 19 unsuspected lesions were imaged; 18 were confirmed by a second diagnostic procedure, and one lesion was not corroborated. A nonspecific uptake of [131]I B72.3 was seen in the left groin and was considered a metastatic lymph node. An aneurysm of the left iliac artery was diagnosed by further investigations, including lymphography, angiography, and CT with and without enhancement. On the other hand,

Table 2 Lesions in 41 Patients with Metastatic Colorectal Cancer Before RIS with Labeled B72.3 MAb

Tumor Site	No. of Lesions	Percentage
Colon recurrence	36	52%
Liver	21	30%
Ascites	5	7%
Peritoneum	5	7%
Other	2	3%

in 18 patients, disease-free on complete clinical workup, no false positive uptake of B72.3 was seen. The two different preparations of B72.3 had a similar sensitivity in the localization of abdominal recurrence and distant metastases: 70% for ^{131}I and 71% for [111]I-labeled B72.3, respectively. Tables 3 and 4 show the results of RIS in these patients in comparison with CT. The RIS with [131]I B72.3 localized 32 solid abdominal tumor nodules, including 24 colonic recurrences and eight peritoneal metastases; missing 12 sites. The peritoneal implants not visualized by RIS had a size > 1 cm at surgery. CT scans detected only 4/10 (40%) peritoneal metastases and 30/34 colonic recurrences. The four missed sites were erroneously diagnosed as postsurgery tissue that localized [131]I B72.3. An example of radiolocalization at an anastomotic site is shown in Figure 2. Unknown distant metastases confined to lungs ($n = 2$) and lymph nodes ($n = 2$) were demonstrated by RIS in four patients considered disease-free according to the clinical workup. Subsequent chest x-ray and CT confirmed these findings. One of the pulmonary metastases was the smallest lesion imaged in our series, measuring 1.2 x 0.8 cm by CT. Both lung metastases became evident in the late images (96 hr) when the background activity in the chest decreased. Ascites, the major cause of CT and US imaging impairment, did not affect RIS. In five patients, discrete peritoneal implants (>5 mm) with concomitant ascitic collection were visualized using [131]I B72.3, as shown in Figure 3.

Further in vitro and cytofluorimetric studies demonstrated that: (1) [131]I was protein-bound, (2) labeled B72.3 was selectively bound to the neoplastic cellular component, and (3) no binding with mesothelial cells, lymphocytes, and macrophages occurred.

Liver represents a critical organ to be evaluated with murine IgGs and with B72.3 labeled with either ^{131}I or ^{111}In, because radioactivity is nonspecifically concentrated and can mask lesions. With iodinated B72.3, 7/16 lesions (44%)

Table 3 Comparative Results in Patients with Metastatic Colorectal Cancer Studied with [131]I B72.3 MAb

Tumor Site	RIS	CT	Unknown
Colon	25[a]/34 (70%)	30/34 (88%)	4[b]
Peritoneum	8/10 (80%)	4/10 (40%)	6
Ascites	5/5 (100%)	5/5 (100%)	–
Liver	7/16 (44%)	16/16 (100%)	–
Other	4/4 (100%)	4/4 (100%)	3

[a]one false positive uptake of [131]I B72.3 due to iliac aneurysm.
[b]unknown lesions detected by RIS and then corroborated by other diagnostic modalities.

Table 4 Comparative Results in Patients with Metastatic Colorectal Cancer Studied with [111]In B72.3 MAb.

Tumor Site	RIS	CT	Unknown
Colon	5/7 (71%)	6/7 (85%)	–
Peritoneum	3/3 (100%)	1/3 (33%)	2
Liver	1/5 (20%)	5/5 (100%)	–
Other	2/2(100%)	2/2 (100%)	2[a]
Total	11/17 (65%)	14/17 (82%)	4

[a]Unknown lesions that were confirmed by CT after RIS.

were detected; in Figure 4 (see color plate after p 66) a metastasis involving the entire left lobe is clearly documented. Using the [111]In B72.3 preparations, only one of the five hepatic metastases was identified owing to nonspecific uptake that was greater than with ^{131}I, perhaps due to transchelation to transferrin.

Results in Tumor Biopsies

IHC was performed on several frozen biopsies from the 19 patients submitted to second-look surgery. In 16 cases, expression of TAG-72 was demonstrated, with an extremely variable pattern. Positive staining corresponded to both viable neoplastic cells and mucin deposits. In nine cases, B72.3 stained more than 80% of the cellular component showing a homogeneous antigenic expression within the tumor nodule; in six cases, the TAG-72 was localized to defined areas, and in four tumors it was expressed by a few foci of viable cells interspersed among normal cells or fibrotic tissue. In all the biopsies with a large mucin component, a strong staining was observed. In a few cases, frozen sections of "normal mucosa" that was removed along with tumors showed a faint positive staining within intracytoplasmic regions and crypta. These in vitro observations led us to review scans to determine whether in vivo false positive uptake of MAb occurred in normal bowel. In our experience, no evidence of B72.3 binding to nonneoplastic tissue was seen.

In seven patients operated on 10 days after the i.v. injection, the percent of ID of [131]I B72.3 bound to tissues was determined by gamma counting and ex vivo quantitative autoradiography. A wide range of binding was observed; in three patients (TAG-72 negative) the levels of ID bound to neoplastic and normal tissues were lower than 0.0001%; in four cases (TAG-72 positive) the range varied from 0.002 to 0.004% of ID per gram of tumor and from 0.0001 to 0.0007% of ID per gram of normal tissues. The tumor/nontumor ratios

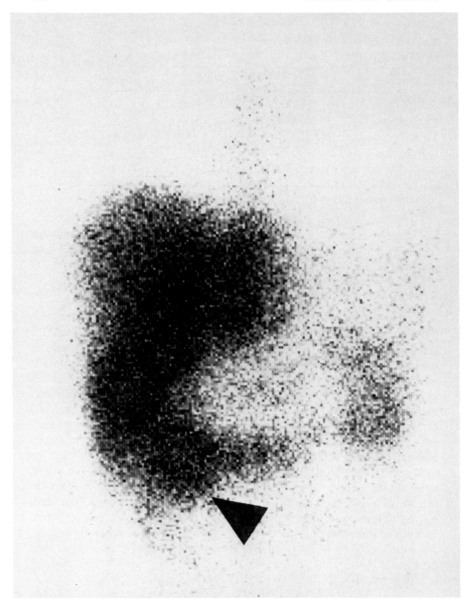

Figure 2 ¹³¹-I B72.3 RIS in a patient followed after resection for colon cancer. Anterior abdominal image at 96 hr showing a focal uptake at anastomotic site (arrowhead). Normal hepatic uptake is seen, and no radioactivity was detectable in the blood pool and in the abdomen.

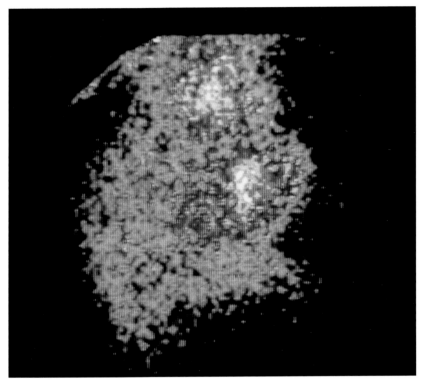

Figure 4 [131]-I B72.3 RIS detects large hepatic metastases involving the left lobe in a patient in follow-up operated for left colonic cancer 36 months earlier.

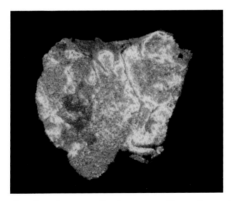

Figure 5 An example of ex vivo quantitative autoradiography performed on a colonic biopsy surgically removed 7 days after the i.v. administration of 4.5 mCi of ^{131}I-B72.3 MAb. The distribution of the antibody reflects the antigenic expression in the section. A necrotic area does not concentrate labeled MAb.

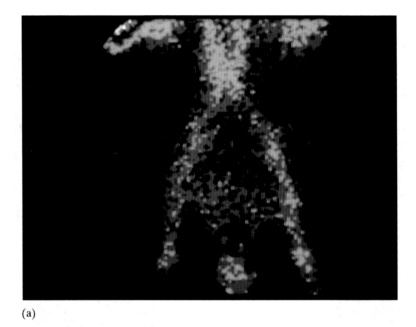

(a)

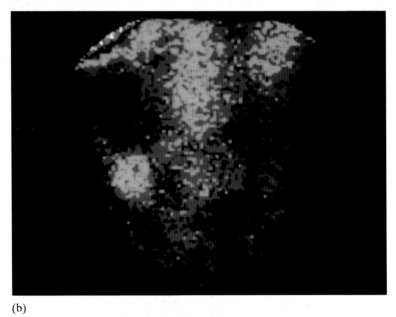

(b)

Figure 6 [111]In B72.3 RIS in recurrent colorectal cancer, anterior abdominal images: (a) 2 hr, (b) 32 hr, (c) subtraction 32 hr minus 2 hr image, (d) reverse subtraction 2 hr minus 32 hr image. The subtraction techniques made it possible to clearly detect the right abdominal recurrence minimizing the background noise; the reverse subtraction shows no blood pool activity in the tumor, confirming the specificity of the tumor targeting.

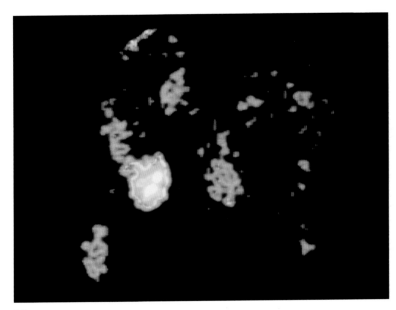

(c)

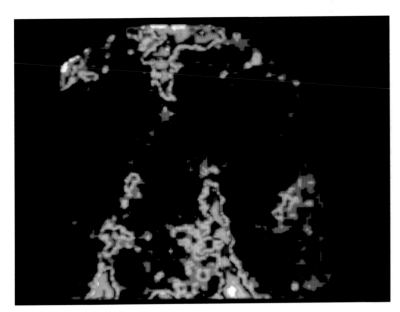

(d)

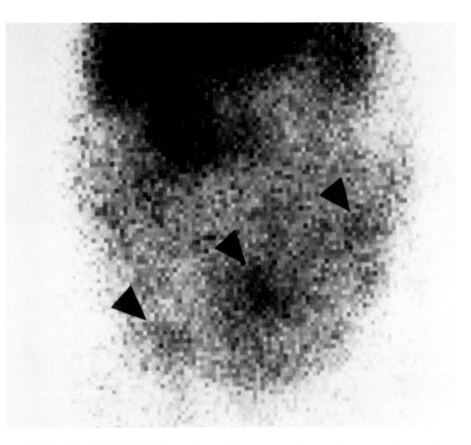

Figure 3 [131]I B72.3 RIS in a patient with recurrent colorectal cancer, ascites, and peritoneal involvement. Anterior view of the abdomen at 72 hr. Foci of uptake (arrowheads) were demonstrated in the left iliac fossa (recurrence) and in peritoneal nodules, which were missed by CT. The diffuse activity in the abdominal cavity is due to ascites.

ranged from 3.5- to 30-fold. By EV-QAR, the [131]I B72.3 distribution within a colonic recurrence is shown in Figure 5 (see color plate after p 66). The heterogeneous distribution of the MAb within the section strongly reflects the heterogeneity of the antigenic expression by neoplastic cells.

DISCUSSION

Evaluation of patients with colon cancer in follow-up after curative surgery represents a critical problem in clinical oncology, because routine procedures underestimate the frequency of tumor recurrences [21]. The results of our study with [131]I B72.3 MAb in 68 patients with primary and metastatic colorectal cancer indicate that RIS has clinical relevance.

In our series 36 patients with recurrent disease (88%) were correctly diagnosed by routine workup; five patients were understaged, and a total of 12 lesions were not identified. Antibody imaging correctly staged 31 patients (75%) as having a metastasis, while in 10 cases (25%) a total of 28 lesions were undetected. In three patients (11 lesions) the IHC performed on several biopsies at second-look surgery demonstrated lack of TAG-72 expression.

The number of lesions seen by B72.3 imaging ($n = 60$) was nearly the same as the number of lesions evaluated by other current diagnostic procedures ($n = 73$). The different imaging modalities were *complementary*: RIS revealed 18 unsuspected lesions that were corroborated by subsequent CT scans or by second-look surgery. The detection of unknown metastases has a great impact in the management of these patients allowing: (1) correct staging and (2) modification of the therapeutic program. In fact, RIS permits a whole-body survey detecting regional and systemic metastases, whereas other imaging procedures examine limited regions or single organs, and their use is mainly based on the onset of clinical symptoms.

The combination of results from clinical workup and RIS accurately staged 39/41 (95%) while the routine practice staged 36/41 (88%) of patients. Two patients were not accurately staged by this combined approach. In nine cases (14%) a drastic change in the therapeutic plan resulted. An overall sensitivity of 68% was obtained for the studies with [131]I B72.3. However, this value increased to 76% if hepatic metastases are not included.

The low sensitivity (>50%) in the detection of primary tumors, at least in the early stages, suggests that this is not a test to use routinely to make the diagnosis of colorectal cancer. It does not improve diagnostic accuracy and sensitivity of other procedures currently used: barium enema, endoscopy, and US. Alternatively, the use of ^{125}I-labeled B72.3 for radioimmunoguided surgery (RIGS) has to be verified in patients with primary and metastatic colorectal cancer. This assumption is related to some properties of B72.3: (1) prolonged in vivo binding at tumor sites over 20 days [22], and (2) high tumor/nontumor ratios (as high as 30-fold) achieved in humans, as we reported in our experience. RIGS with [125]I B72.3 is currently used by several groups [23] to detect "subclinical" (<5 mm) or "unknown" lesions, with promising results, although the 14-to-20-day interval between MAb administration and RIGS still represents the main limitation for diffusion of this technique.

A clinical issue that needs to be resolved is the timing of performance of either RIGS or RIS in patients during follow-up. Using B72.3, the study can be programmed while monitoring the circulating TAG-72 every 3–6 months. In our experience (unpublished data), circulating levels of TAG-72 increase significantly in patients with large tumors or wide disease spread and in mucinous histotypes of gastrointestinal tumors. Normal levels of circulating TAG-72 do not exclude that recurrences and/or metastases have occurred; in eight patients in our series with normal TAG-72, RIS with labeled B72.3 demonstrated tumor masses.

The analysis of radioimmunoscintigraphic studies requires well-trained physicians to obtain and integrate all the information (pharmacokinetics and imaging) and to evaluate whether tumor is visualized. The background in the blood pool and some organs can negatively affect RIS imaging. To overcome this problem, subtraction techniques have been introduced. We used the subtraction of early images from later ones with very satisfactory results, as shown in Figure 6 (see color plate after p 66). However, for the routine clinical use of labeled MAbs, isotopes with a shorter half-life (i.e., ^{99m}Tc, ^{123}I, etc.), and single-photon emission tomography (SPECT) may be more suitable approaches.

Innovations directly or indirectly related to B72.3 need to be mentioned for the impact they may have in the management of patients with colon cancer using the radioimmunological approach for both diagnostic and therapeutic purposes. The use of second-generation MAbs [24], such as CC49, that have a greater affinity constant for TAG-72 than B72.3 should favor the percentage of ID bound to the tumor. The development of recombinant/chimeric B72.3 (chB72.3) [25], which shows the same pattern of reactivity as the native B72.3, may allow repeated injections of MAb in the same patients, minimizing the production of HAMA and the related risks and permitting a wider use of RIS in follow-up. The development of new chelates for metallic isotopes such as ^{99m}Tc and ^{111}In, which ensure a greater in vivo stability of the labeled immunoreagents, should favor the use of these isotopes which are more suitable for gamma imaging.

The evidence that TAG-72 can be up-regulated by some biological response modifiers, such as recombinant alpha and gamma interferons [26], opens new horizons in tumor targeting for diagnostic and therapeutic purposes. Specific binding should be significantly improved by the increase of the antigenic molar content at tumor sites.

In conclusion, B72.3 tumor targeting in colorectal cancer is a safe and sensitive procedure that is able to identify patients with metastatic disease. B72.3 RIS should be used in patients with suspected recurrent colon cancer and in patients with large primary tumors to detect unknown or distant metastases that are clinically asymptomatic.

REFERENCES

1. Kholer G, Milstein C. Continuous cultures of fused cells secreting antibody of predefined specificity. Nature (London) 1975; 256:495–7.

2. Larson SM, Brown JP, Wright PW, Carrasquillo JA, Hellstrom I, Hellstrom KE. Imaging of melanoma with I-131-labeled monoclonal antibodies. J Nucl Med 1983; 23:123–9.

3. Epenetos AA, Munro AJ, Stewart S, Rampling R, Lambert HE, et al. Antibody-guided irradiation of advanced ovarian cancer with intraperitoneally administered radiolabeled monoclonal antibodies. J Clin Oncol 1987; 5:1890–9.

4. Mach JP, Buchegger F, Forni M, Ritschard J, Berche C, Lumbroso MD, et al. Use of radiolabeled monoclonal anti-CEA antibodies for the detection of human carcinomas by external photoscanning and tomoscintigraphy. Immunol Today 1981; 2:239–49.

5. Goldenberg DM, Deland F, Kim EE, Bennet SJ, et al. Use of radiolabeled antibodies to carcinoembryonic antigen for the detection and localization of diverse cancer by external photoscanning. N Engl J Med 1978; 298:1384–8.

6. Mach JP, Chatal JF, Lumbroso JD, et al. Tumor localization in patients by radiolabeled monoclonal antibodies against colon carcinoma. Cancer Res 1983; 43:5593–5600.

7. Johnson VG, Schlom J, Peterson A, Bennet J, Magnani JL, Colcher D. Analysis of a human tumor-associated glycoprotein (TAG-72) identified by monoclonal antibody B72.3. Cancer Res 1986; 46:850–7.

8. Ohuchi N, Thor A, Nose M, Fujita J, Kyogoku M, Schlom J. Tumor-associated glycoprotein (TAG-72) detected in adenocarcinomas and benign lesions of the stomach. Int J Cancer 1986; 38:643–50.

9. Thor A, Gorstein F, Ohuchi N, Szpack CA, Johnston WW, Schlom J. Tumor-associated glycoprotein (TAG-72) in ovarian carcinomas defined by monoclonal antibody B72.3. J Natl Cancer Inst 1986; 76:995–1006.

10. Thor A, Viglione MJ, Muraro R, Ohuchi N, Schlom J, Gorstein F. Monoclonal antibody B72.3 reactivity with human endometrium: a study of normal and malignant tissues. Int J Gynecol Pathol. 1987; 6(3):235–47.

11. Renda A, Salvatore M, Sava M, Landi R, Lastoria S, Coppola L, et al. Immunoscintigraphy in the follow-up of patients operated for carcinoma of the sigmoid and rectum. Preliminary report with a new monoclonal antibody:B72.3. Dis Colon Rectum 1987; 30(9)683–6.

12. Colcher D, Esteban JM, Carrasquillo JA, Sugarbaker P, Reynolds JC, Bryant G, Larson SM, Schlom J. Quantitative analyses of selective radiolabeled monoclonal antibody localization in metastatic lesions of colorectal cancer patients. Cancer Res 1987; 47:1185–9.

13. Colcher d, Carrasquillo JA, Esteban JM, Sugarbaker P, Reynolds JC, Siler K, Bryant G, Larson S, Schlom J. Radiolabeled monoclonal antibody B72.3 localization in metastatic lesions of colorectal cancer patients. Nucl Med Biol 1987; 14(3):251–62.

14. Lastoria S, D'Amico P, Mansi L, Giordano GG, Rossiello R, et al. A prospective imaging study of I-131 B72.3 monoclonal antibody in patients with epithelial ovarian cancer: preliminary report. Nucl Med Commun 1988; 9:347–56.

15. Colcher D, Horan Hand P, Nuti M, Schlom J. A spectrum of monoclonal antibodies reactive with human mammary tumor cells. Proc Natl Acad Sci USA 1981; 78:3199–3203.

16. Stramignoni D, Bowen R, Atkinson BF, Schlom J. Differential reactivity of monoclonal antibodies with human colon adenocarcinomas and adenomas. Int J Cancer 1983; 31:543–52.

17. Fraker PJ, Speck JC. Protein and cell membrane iodinations with a sparingly soluble chloramide. 1,3,4,6-tetrachloro-3a,6a-diphenylglycouril. Biochem Biophys Res Commun 1978; 80:849–57.

18. Hnatowich DJ, Layne WW, Childs RL. The preparation and labelling of DTPA coupled albumin. Int J Appl Radiat Isotope 1982; 33:327–32.

19. Granowska M, Shepherd J, Britton KE et al. Ovarian cancer diagnosis using I-123 monoclonal antibody in comparison with surgical findings. Nucl Med Commun 1984; 5:485–99.

20. Hsu SM, Raine L, Fauger H. Use of avidin-biotin peroxidase complex (ABC) in immunoperoxidase technique: a comparison between ABC and unlabeled antibody PAP procedures. J Hist Cytochem 1981; 29:577–80.

21. Gilbert JM, Jeffrey I, Evan M, Mark AE. Sites of recurrent tumor after curative colorectal surgery: implications for adjuvant therapy. Br J Surg. 1984; 71:203–5.

22. Colcher D, Keenan AM, Larson SM, Schlom J. Prolonged binding of a radiolabeled monoclonal antibody (B72.3) used for in situ radioimmunodetection of human colon carcinoma xenografts. Cancer Res 1984; 44:5744–51.

23. Martin EW, Mojzisik CM, Hinkle GM, et al. Radioimmunoguided surgery using monoclonal antibody. Am J Surg 1988; 156:386–92.

24. Muraro R, Kuroki M, Wunderlich D, Poole DJ, Colcher D, Thor A, et al. Generation and characterization of B72.3 second generation monoclonal antibodies reactive with tumor-associated glycoprotein 72 antigen. Cancer Res 1988; 48:4588–96.

25. Colcher D, Milenic D, Roselli M, et al. Characterization and biodistribution of recombinant and recombinant/chimeric constructs of monoclonal antibody B72.3. Cancer Res 1989; 49:1738–45.

26. Guadagni F, Schlom J, Johnston WW, Szpak CA, Goldstein D, et al. Selective interferon-induced enhancement of tumor-associated antigens on a spectrum of freshly isolated human adenocarcinoma cells. J Natl Cancer Inst 1989; 81(7):502–12.

5

Multicenter Clinical Trials of Monoclonal Antibody B72.3-GYK-DTPA ^{111}In (^{111}In-CYT-103; OncoScint CR103) in Patients with Colorectal Carcinoma

Hani H. Abdel-Nabi and Ralph J. Doerr
State University of New York at Buffalo, Buffalo, New York

INTRODUCTION

The American Cancer Society estimated that 110,000 new colon cancer cases and 45,000 new rectal cancer cases would be diagnosed in the United States in 1990, with an average of 53,300 and 7,600 deaths from colon and rectum cancers, respectively [1]. The stage of colorectal cancer at the time of initial diagnosis is the most important prognostic determinant. Currently existing conventional imaging modalities, particularly computerized axial tomography (CT), cannot adequately stage tumors, because they are limited in their ability to determine the extent of tumor invasion into the bowel wall, nor can they determine metastatic involvement of lymph nodes [2–5] the two essential criteria used in the Dukes Staging System [6]. Several recent clinical studies have demonstrated the usefulness of radiolabeled monoclonal antibodies in the imaging of patients with colorectal carcinoma [7–16]. A preliminary clinical trial was performed with the anti-TAG-72 murine monoclonal antibody (B72.3) labeled with ^{111}In after site-specific conjugation to the antibody oligosaccharide moiety with the linker-chelator glycyltyrosyl-(N-ϵ-diethylenetriaminepenta-acetic acid)-lysine (GYK-DTPA). Antibody images were positive in 37 of 50 patients (74%) with either primary or recurrent colorectal carcinoma following single intravenous infusions of 0.2, 1, 2, or 20 mg of the radiolabeled antibody conjugate CYT-103 (B72.3-GYK-DTPA) [17]. In two subsequent pilot studies, we reported that tumor detection with ^{111}In-CYT-103 was generally independent of the dose of conjugated antibody used [18], although improvement in targeting of primary colorectal carcinomas occurred when a 1.0-mg dose of monoclonal antibody (MAb) was used (detection rate = 75%), compared to a dose of 0.5 mg of conjugated MAb (detection rate = 20%) [19]. With this information in mind, a pivotal prospective multi-institutional trial was conducted to evaluate the sensitivity, specificity, and accuracy of ^{111}In-CYT-103 imaging in presurgical colorectal carcinoma patients. Another objective of this study was to assess the impact of ^{111}In-CYT-103 imaging on the clinical management of these patients, and this will be the subject of a subsequent chapter.

^{111}In-CYT-103 IMAGING; THE MULTI-INSTITUTIONAL TRIAL

This report describes the methods and results of a prospective, multi-institutional clinical trial evaluating the performance (sensitivity, specificity, and accuracy) of ^{111}In-CYT-103 immunoscintigraphy in detecting primary and recurrent colorectal tumors, including occult lesions, in 103 presurgical patients.

Design and Statistical Consideration

This was an open-label, nonrandomized trial to determine the performance and efficacy of ^{111}In-CYT-103 immunoscintigraphy in colorectal carcinoma patients. Imaging performance was determined by comparing the results of MAb image interpretation (prospective and retrospective) with the surgical and histopathological findings for each patient.

Patient Selection

Patients enrolled in this study were presurgical patients with a tissue diagnosis of either primary or recurrent colorectal carcinoma, or with a high clinical or radiological suspicion of primary or recurrent tumors. Patient performance status on the Karnofsky scale was usually above 60%, and expected survival was 2 months or more. Also, patients must not have received conventional or investigational antitumor therapy for at least 4 weeks prior to MAb infusion to prevent superimposition of possible adverse reactions, and also to minimize potential, unexpected interactions between antitumor therapy and ^{111}In-CYT-103 immunoscintigraphy. Patients with antitumor therapy–related toxicities were enrolled only if they had recovered from prior toxicity.

In the initial phase of the trial, patients with low hemoglobin (≤ 10 g/dl), low hematocrit ($< 30\%$), white blood count less than $3000/\mu l$, or platelet count less than $100,000/\mu l$, as well as those with poor renal function (creatinine > 2 mg/dl), were excluded. These exclusion criteria were dropped after ascertainment of the safety of single intravenous infusions of 1.0 mg CYT-103. Also excluded were patients who had received a prior injection of murine monoclonal antibodies.

Demographic Characteristics

Of the 103 evaluable patients enrolled in this trial, 62 were men and 41 were women, ranging in age from 37 to 88 years (mean = 65 years). Sixty-one patients were being evaluated for primary colorectal carcinoma, while 42 patients were evaluated for recurrent cancer. The majority of primary tumors were located in the left colon, predominantly sigmoid colon, rectum, and descending colon. All patients had to provide written informed consent. The study protocol was approved by the institutional review board of each of 23 participating centers.

Baseline Evaluation

Prior to infusion, each patient had a complete evaluation, which included a medical history with particular reference to previous murine MAb exposure, a physical examination, a complete blood count with differential and platelet count, liver and kidney function tests, and routine urinalysis. These tests were repeated within 5–7 days of CYT-103 infusion. Baseline serum carcinoembryonic antigen (CEA) and TAG-72 levels were measured with commercially available kits. Serum titers of human antimouse antibodies (HAMA) were measured using the Immustrip HAMA Test System (Immunomedics, Warren, NJ), a direct enzyme-linked immunosorbent assay [15]. HAMA titers less than 0.4 μg/ml were considered negative. The development of HAMA was assessed in serial serum samples obtained 2–8 weeks postinfusion.

Baseline chest x-rays and computed tomography (CT) scans of the abdomen and pelvis were performed on all patients prior to surgery.

¹¹¹In-CYT-103 Administration

Upon completion of the baseline evaluations, patients were given a single intravenous dose of 1.0 mg of CYT-103 labeled with 4.21 ± 0.68 (mean ± SD) mCi of ¹¹¹In. Radiolabeled antibody conjugate was prepared by adding a buffered solution of approximately 5.5 mCi of ¹¹¹In Cl_3 to the vial containing the CYT-103 dose. The contents of the vial were gently mixed and incubated at room temperature for 30 min. The percentage of ¹¹¹In bound to CYT-103 was tested using an instant thin-layer chromatography procedure. Details of the radiolabeling procedure have been described previously [17,19]. ¹¹¹In-CYT-103 was administered by slow bolus push over approximately 5 min.

^{111}In-CYT-Scintigraphy

Planar scintiscans, including anterior and posterior projections of the thorax, abdomen, and pelvis, were obtained using large field-of-view cameras fitted with parallel-hole, medium-energy collimators and adjusted to both ^{111}In photon peaks (173 and 247 Kev) with a 20% window. Images of 10^6 counts or 10 min, whichever occurred first, were obtained on two separate occasions at least 24 hr apart, usually between 2 and 5 days post ^{111}In-CYT-103 infusion. Nuclear medicine data were acquired in a digital format in a 128 x 128 matrix and stored on a track reel-to-reel magnetic tape or soft-sectored floppy disks. The abdomen and pelvis were also evaluated by emission computed tomography (SPECT), usually between 2 and 5 days postinfusion. Extra-abdominal areas that were suspicious for tumor on planar scans were also evaluated by SPECT. Most clinical sites used single-headed systems, and acquisition parameters included a 360° rotating orbit, sampling every 6 degrees with an approximately 40 sec acquisition per stop. A filtered back-projection algorithm was used for tomographic reconstruction.

Rigorous gamma camera quality control was maintained throughout the trial. For planar imaging, intrinsic ^{111}In flood and bar phantoms (minimum 2 x 10^6 counts) were acquired prior to the first imaging session for each patient.

Extrinsic floods with a medium-energy collimator using either [57]Co source or ^{99m}Tc flood source were acquired prior to study initiation and then on a weekly basis.

Quality control of the SPECT imaging systems included a 30-million-count extrinsic uniformity correction, center-of-rotation determination, linearity, and patient motion detection (sinogram display). Either an ^{111}In fillable phantom or a [57]Co disc source was used for uniformity correction. An ^{111}In point source was used for COR correction. These quality control procedures were performed prior to study initiation and weekly thereafter or whenever needed.

^{111}In-CYT-103 Scan Interpretation

The on-site nuclear medicine physician interpreted the scans prospectively with the results of the other presurgical tests (CT scans, chest x-rays, barium enema, colonoscopy, magnetic resonance imaging, and liver-spleen scans) available for each patient.

Abnormal scan findings were mapped on an anatomical drawing and discussed, along with the results of other presurgical tests, with the surgeon preoperatively. In most cases, surgery was performed within 2 weeks after completion of the two imaging sessions. During surgery, an attempt was made to evaluate all known lesions as well as new lesions indicated by ^{111}In-CYT-103 imaging. When appropriate, biopsies of these unsuspected lesions were obtained.

All resected tissues were examined by standard histopathological techniques and graded according to a modified Dukes classification. TAG-72 expression in resected tumor specimens was determined using the avidin-biotin-immunoperoxidase method [20,21], which was performed in a central, specialized laboratory.

^{111}In-CYT-103 Performance

The performance of ^{111}In-CYT-103 immunoscintigraphy during this trial was assessed by comparing the antibody imaging findings for each patient with the surgical and histopathological findings. Two separate performance evaluations of ^{111}In-CYT-103 scintigraphy were made: one based on the prospective interpretation of the antibody scan by the unblinded nuclear medicine physician at each clinical site, and the other based on the retrospective interpretation by two independent blinded nuclear medicine experts. Each of these evaluations will be described in detail in the following sections.

Sensitivity, Specificity, and Accuracy

Surgical and histopathological results showed that 92 of 103 patients studied had colorectal carcinoma, and 10 patients were free of disease. One additional patient evaluated for recurrent colorectal carcinoma was found to have a second primary malignancy (small cell carcinoma of the lung) and was excluded from the tabulations of ^{111}In-CYT-103 imaging performance parameters, which are listed in Table 1. In the 92 patients with surgically confirmed disease, ^{111}In-CYT-103 imaging detected 82 of 126 confirmed carcinoma lesions. In addition, 33 other lesions were detected and were considered highly suggestive of and compatible with malignancies related to the primary colorectal carcinomas. Only five of these lesions could be evaluated histopathologically, and none were found to be malignant. Three of these five false positive findings were inflammatory lesions, one was a tubulovillous adenoma, and one was normal tissue that did not contain TAG-72. The mechanisms behind the false positive MAb accumulation in nonmalignant tissues not expressing or containing the antigen(s) against which the MAb is raised are not clearly understood. However, MAb accumulation in nonmalignant tissues, especially lymph nodes that contained CEA by immunohistochemistry, has previously been reported [22]. These ^{111}In MAb-positive, tumor-free nodes were usually in the draining pathway of the original or primary tumor.

Twenty-eight of the thirty-three unconfirmed radiolocalizations were not biopsied and are therefore considered indeterminate findings. Of these, 17 were within the surgical field, and the remaining 11 were outside the field of surgery. Follow-up diagnostic procedures confirmed the results of the antibody scans in six patients with seven indeterminate lesions, likely to represent

Table 1 ^{111}In-CYT-103 Imaging Performance Characteristics of 102 Evaluable Patients

Patient population	Performance parameters	% and number of patients correctly identified by MAb imaging	
		Prospective (on-site readers)	Retrospective (blinded readers)
Patient with surgically confirmed tumors	Sensitivity	69.6% (64/92)	59.2%
Patients with no tumors at surgery	Specificity	90.0% (9/10)	85%
All available patient	Accuracy	71.6% (73/103)	61.7%

metastatic adenocarcinoma to bone (four lesions), liver (one lesion), retroperitoneal lymph nodes (one lesion), and brain (one lesion). Four of the seven indeterminate lesions were initially identified by ^{111}In-CYT-103 imaging and subsequently confirmed by bone scans, CT, or magnetic resonance imaging (MRI).

Occult Disease

In five patients with primary colorectal cancer, ^{111}In-CYT-103 immunoscintigraphy detected additional tumor lesions that were not suspected by physical examination or other presurgical diagnostic tests conducted prior to antibody imaging. Antibody scans detected more extensive disease in one patient, carcinomatosis in one patient, and bony metastasis in the third patient. Primary lesions in the rectosigmoid and sigmoid colon were initially detected in the other two patients.

^{111}In-CYT-103 MAb scans detected occult disease in six patients with recurrent colorectal carcinoma, three of whom had elevated serum CEA levels and otherwise negative presurgical workup. These lesions were surgically and histopathologically confirmed as true positive localizations. Four patients had negative MAb scans and negative exploratory surgery. Immunoscintigraphy did not detect metastatic involvement of the right lobe of the liver in three patients with elevated CEA levels, one of whom also had a rectosigmoid carcinoma also missed by ^{111}In-CYT-103. False positive localization in inflammatory tissue in the mesentery was also found in that patient. These data, as well as our own experience [23], suggest that antibody imaging has value in detecting occult disease outside the liver and in confirming concurrent negative diagnostic evaluations in patients presenting with elevated serum CEA levels.

Although considered to be valuable for screening for postoperative recurrences, elevated serum CEA levels have been shown to be falsely elevated in approximately 30% of patients [24]. Also, recurrences have been found during second-look surgery in symptomatic patients who did not have elevated CEA levels [25–27].

Immunoscintigraphy with ^{111}In-CYT-103 has been able to confirm the absence of distant disease in 18 of 22 patients with isolated recurrences, and this could have a major impact on the decision to surgically explore these patients [28,29]. Thus, antibody imaging may be particularly useful as a presurgical diagnostic test for a subset of patients with presumed isolated recurrences by allowing more definitive treatment in those with localized, resectable tumors.

Liver Metastases

^{111}In-CYT-103 immunoscintigraphy detected liver metastases in 21 of 38 patients (sensitivity = 55.3%). However, the majority of these liver lesions were seen as photopenic areas or "cold defects." ^{111}In-CYT-103 sensitivity for liver metastases would be considerably lower if we consider only hot lesions as true positive findings. The low detection rate of ^{111}In-CYT-103 imaging for liver lesions could be attributed to the high liver background due to the nonspecific accumulation of free or chelate-bound ^{111}In or ^{111}In antibody conjugate, which results in the visualization of liver metastases as photopenic or cold defects. Attempts to decrease the amount of liver uptake of ^{111}In-CYT-103 by the administration of larger doses of antibody either concurrently or prior to the radiolabeled conjugate have not been effective [19], as opposed to a positive dose-response relationship between detection of "hot" liver lesions and increasing amounts of ^{111}In-labeled anti-CEA antibody ZCE 025 [10,14,15]. As previously reported, a variety of histological and immunohistochemical factors affect radiolabeled antibody localization in liver metastases [19]. For example, tumors with moderate to excessive amounts of necrosis, those which are poorly to moderately well differentiated, those with no or poor antigenic expression, and those measuring 2.5 cm or more have a tendency to appear as cold defects. Thus, visualization of liver metastases as cold defects may relate to local and intrinsic factors, and not to failure of the technique itself.

Factors Affecting Imaging Performance

Other factors that could affect the performance of ^{111}In-CYT-103 immunoscinti-graphy, such as level of circulating TAG-72 in serum, tumor content of TAG–72 and its cellular expression, and previous antitumor therapy, will be discussed.

Serum Levels of TAG-72 Antigen

Of the 82 patients with surgically confirmed adenocarcinoma and evaluable serum samples, 20 (24.4%) had positive TAG-72 serum titers ($\geq$10 U/ml) prior to ^{111}In-CYT-103 administration. A slight increase in imaging sensitivity was seen in patients with positive (85.0%) versus negative (62.9%) serum TAG-72 levels. These findings are consistent with the imaging data reported by Carrasquillo et al. for ^{131}I-labeled MAb B72.3 [12].

Tumor Expression of TAG-72 Antigen

Eighty-eight of 126 surgically confirmed adenocarcinoma lesions were evaluated immunohistochemically for the expression of TAG-72. ^{111}In-CYT-103 immunoscintigraphy was positive in 10 of 21 (47.6%) patients with tumors that contained TAG-72 in <5% of tumor cells per specimen lesion, whereas an increase in lesion detectability was observed in tumors expressing TAG-72 in 5–50% of cells (31 of 48 patients positive, sensitivity = 64.6%) and those which expressed TAG-72 in $\geq$50% of tumor cells (15 of 19 patients positive, sensitivity = 78.9%). The increase in sensitivity of [111]In-CYT-103 imaging for tumor lesions expressing the antigen in less than 5% versus those with 5% or more cells staining positive with immunohistochemistry was statistically significant ($p = 0.04$), and is consistent with earlier data reported for this antibody conjugate, administered at various dose levels [17,19].

Effect of Prior Antitumor Therapy on Imaging Performance

Chemotherapy and radiation therapy have the potential to affect tumor antigenic expression and could therefore alter subsequent successful ^{111}In-CYT-103 immunoscintigraphy [30]. Twenty patients enrolled in this trial had received radiation, chemotherapy, or immunotherapy prior to ^{111}In-CYT-103 administration. In this study, the performance of ^{111}In-CYT-103 immunoscintigraphy was similar among patients who had prior chemo- and radiation therapy and those who did not (Table 2).

Contribution of SPECT to Antibody Imaging Performance

The effect of SPECT on ^{111}In-CYT-103 imaging performance was determined by comparing the blinded readers' interpretations of planar and planar plus SPECT images for each patient. Eighty-five of the 92 patients with proven adenocarcinomas had both planar and SPECT imaging performed according to the image acquisition protocol described earlier. SPECT increased ^{111}In-CYT-103 imaging sensitivity from 55.3% to 61.2% for one reader and from 50.6% to 58.8% for the other reader. The incremental effect of SPECT on imaging sensitivity was statistically significant for one reader ($p = 0.02$), but

Table 2 Relationship Between Prior Antitumor Therapy and Performance of ^{111}In-CYT-103

Per-patient imaging performance parameter	Previous antitumor therapy	No previous antitumor therapy
Sensitivity	68.4% (13/19)	69.9% (51/73)
Specificity	100% (1/1)	88.9% (8/9)
Accuracy	70.0% (14/20)	72.0% (59/82)

not the other. Modest incremental increases in tumor detection rates with SPECT imaging have previously been described with ^{111}In-CYT-103 and other ^{111}In-labeled MAbs [10,11,15,16]. However, SPECT also provides for better tumor definition and anatomical localization and could perhaps be utilized to estimate the tumor volume. In particular, SPECT could be helpful in delineating small (less than 1.5 cm) liver lesions and in separating bladder activity from that present in a pelvic tumor [19]. Rigorous quality control methods should be adopted when SPECT acquisition is desired, and the nuclear

Table 3 Performance of ^{111}In-CYT-103 and CT Imaging in Patients with Primary Colorectal Carcinomas[a]

Per-patient imaging performance parameters	^{111}In-CYT-103 Immunoscintigraphy	CT scanning
Sensitivity	69.4% (59/85)	65.9% (56/85)
Specificity	88.9% (8/9)	88.9% (8/9)
Accuracy	71.3% (67/94)	68.1% (65/94)

[a]Comparison based on patients who had both antibody imaging and CT scanning prior to surgery.

CYT-103-¹¹¹IN
MULTICENTER EFFICACY TRIALS
CT Comparison

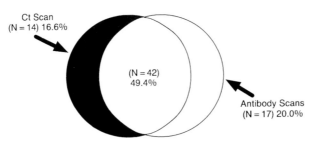

Figure 1 Populations of patients with colorectal adenocarcinoma who were correctly diagnosed by MAb and CT imaging were overlapping but were not identical.

Table 4 Comparison of the Sensitivities of ¹¹¹In-CYT-103 and CT Imaging for Lesions Located in the Pelvis, Liver, and Other Sites

	Sensitivity	
Lesion location	¹¹¹In-CYT-103	CT scanning
Pelvis	68.9% (32/45)	59.0%[a] (23/39)
Liver	55.3% (21/38)	86.5%[a] (32/37)
Other	69.8% (30/43)	47.5%[a] (19/40)

[a] CT scanning showed statistically significant ($p = 0.01$) differences in tumor detection rates for liver lesions versus extrahepatic (i.e., pelvic, other) lesions.

medicine physician should familiarize himself with SPECT techniques and interpretation in the abdomen and pelvis before a real incremental effect on tumor detection with SPECT will be observed.

Data obtained from this trial and an earlier one [31] suggest that the optimal imaging time with ^{111}In-CYT-103 is between 2 and 3 days after administration. Reducing the time interval between MAb administration and completion of the imaging studies to less than a week will undeniably make this procedure more attractive to the surgeon or medical oncologist who wishes to evaluate the patient prior to instituting definitive therapy.

Comparison of ^{111}In-CYT-103 Imaging Performance and CT in Colorectal Carcinoma Patients

Although ^{111}In-CYT-103 multicenter imaging trials were not designed as controlled comparative studies with CT imaging, analysis of the data revealed some interesting information. CT scanning was selected for comparison because it is commonly performed in the routine presurgical workup of primary and recurrent colorectal carcinoma patients.

In 85 patients with surgically confirmed adenocarcinomas, the sensitivity, specificity, and accuracy of ^{111}In-CYT-103 and CT scanning were numerically similar (Table 3). However, immunoscintigraphy correctly identified tumor lesions in 17 patients with negative CT scans, while CT imaging identified tumors in 14 patients with negative MAb scans. When the two diagnostic modalities were used in combination, tumor lesions were correctly identified in 73 of 85 patients (86%). These results indicate that the value of ^{111}In-CYT-103 and CT scanning in preoperative detection of lesions can be enhanced when used in a complementary fashion (Fig. 1).

A difference was noted in the performance of ^{111}In-CYT-103 and CT scanning when lesion location was evaluated separately. The data presented in Table 4 are consistent with the published findings for the relative sensitivities of CT imaging in the pelvis, the liver, and other (primarily abdominal) lesions in colorectal cancer patients. Antibody imaging detected a greater percentage of lesions in the pelvis (68.9% versus 59.0%) and in other areas (69.8% versus 47.5%), and CT imaging detected a greater proportion of liver lesions (86.5% versus 55.3%).

There was no statistically significant difference in antibody imaging for extrahepatic lesions versus liver lesions ($p = 0.26$); however, the sensitivity of CT imaging was significantly lower ($p = 0.01$) for extrahepatic lesions than for lesions located in the liver.

The difference in the performance of antibody and CT imaging with respect to the location of the tumor lesions provides an explanation for the enhanced sensitivity and accuracy observed when these two imaging modalities are used in a complementary manner.

SAFETY AND HAMA RESPONSE

Seven patients experienced a total of nine adverse reactions that were considered possibly related to the murine MAb administration. The most frequent adverse reactions included fever and itching, each experienced by three patients. In addition, one patient each developed mild hypertension, queasiness, and angioedema. All these adverse reactions resolved either spontaneously or with appropriate medications. None of these reactions was considered serious, and no biochemical side effects from the ^{111}In-CYT-103 administration were reported during this trial. The low rate of adverse reactions (6%) and their mildness is in accordance with our previous experience and those of others with B72.3 [12,13] or other MAbs [9–11] and is further documentation of the safety of single intravenous infusion of murine monoclonal antibodies.

The presence of HAMA was evaluated in serum samples obtained from 95 patients, both prior to and at 2, 4, and 8 weeks postinfusion. Positive postinfusion HAMA titers were found in the sera of 31 patients (33%) and were not associated with an increased incidence of adverse reactions, nor did they interfere with positive ^{111}In-CYT-103 tumor detection. The incidence of HAMA formation following a single intravenous infusion of 1.0 mg of CYT-103 is slightly lower than that reported with MAb B72.3 labeled with ^{131}I [12].

SUMMARY AND CONCLUSION

The results of this clinical trial involving 23 sites indicated that ^{111}In-CYT-103 immunoscintigraphy identified 70% of all patients with surgically confirmed disease when interpreted by the on-site physician. The sensitivity of ^{111}In-CYT-103 imaging was slightly lower when interpreted retrospectively by the blinded readers in the absence of any patient-specific information. ^{111}In-CYT-103 imaging sensitivity was similar in patients with primary and recurrent disease, but lower for liver metastases than for extrahepatic disease. Thirty-three previously unknown lesions were visualized by immunoscintigraphy; tissue confirmation was available for only five lesions, and all were found to be free of tumor. Only one of the lesions evaluated was TAG-72 positive. Twenty-eight lesions were outside the surgical field or not biopsied. Although no tissue confirmation was available, seven (25%) of these lesions were identified as consistent with metastatic disease by other conventional modalities. Importantly, antibody scans detected occult tumor lesions in 11 of the 92 patients with surgically confirmed adenocarcinoma, and accurately diagnosed 7 of 10 patients with elevated serum CEA levels and negative conventional workup. Surgery confirmed the presence of tumor identified only by ^{111}In-CYT-103 in three patients, while four patients with negative scans had no evidence of recurrent disease at surgery. Antibody scans confirmed the absence of additional disease in 18 of 22 patients with isolated hepatic or pelvic recurrences in whom curative surgery was contemplated. The results of this multicenter trial suggest that CYT-103 immunoscintigraphy can provide information that is complementary to that derived from standard diagnostic techniques. During the workup of patients with primary colorectal carcinoma, this modality assesses the entire body and allows for the identification of multiple lesions at various locations simultaneously. It can then redirect attention and further workup to those areas not originally surveyed. Of special interest in this regard is the identification of occult lesions in five patients with primary colorectal cancer.

^{111}In-CYT-103 imaging was found superior to CT in the localization of primary colorectal cancer, but neither modality could adequately assess the extent of tumor penetration through the bowel wall (the T stage in the TNM system) or the N status. The limitations of CT in evaluating T and N are well documented, and the limitations of ^{111}In-based immunoscintigraphy for these same lesions have recently been described [11,19]. Another limitation of ^{111}In-CYT-103 immunoscintigraphy is in the identification of liver metastases. Although the reported sensitivity of ^{111}In-CYT-103 imaging of liver metastases in this trial is 55%, most of these lesions were seen as cold defects. Thus, CT remains the modality of choice in evaluating metastatic liver disease in patients prior to surgery.

However, ^{111}In-CYT-103 imaging provided diagnostically useful information in the workup of patients with elevated serum CEA levels and no radiographic evidence of recurrence as well as in patients with localized recurrent disease who are surgical candidates. In the former group, ^{111}In-CYT-103 immunoscintigraphy should be used prior to other standard diagnostic techniques, which have well-documented limitations in screening for occult disease [32,33]. The ability to more accurately assess the extent of disease locally and outside the abdomen in patients with localized recurrence is important, as a potentially curative procedure may be undertaken [28,29,34]. Alternatively, the identification of unresectable disease may result in selection of other therapy, such as radiation or chemotherapy. The low incidence of adverse reactions and HAMA formation following single intravenous infusions of 1.0 mg CYT-103 conjugated to ^{111}In, combined with its demonstrated ability to detect 70% of primary and recurrent tumors, including occult lesions, suggests a clinically useful role for ^{111}In-CYT-103 immunoscintigraphy in the workup of colorectal carcinoma patients prior to surgery.

REFERENCES

1. Cancer Statistics 1990. CA 1990; 40:18–9.
2. Freeny PC, Marks WM, Ryan JA, Bolen JW. Colorectal carcinoma evaluation with CT: preoperative staging and detection of post-operative recurrence. Radiology 1986; 158:347–53.
3. Thompson WM, Halvorsen RA, Forster WL Jr, Roberts L, Gibbons R. Preoperative and postoperative CT staging of rectosigmoid carcinoma. Am J Radiol 1988; 146:703–10.
4. Thompson WM, Halvorsen RA Jr. Computed tomographic staging of gastrointestinal malignancies. II. The small bowel, colon and rectum. Invest Radiol 1987; 22:96–105.
5. Kelvin FM, Maglinte DDT. Colorectal carcinoma: a radiologic and clinical review. Radiology 1987; 164:1–8.
6. Dukes CE. The classification of cancer of the rectum. J Pathol 1983; 35:323–32.
7. Berche C, Mach JP, Lumbroso JD, et al. Tomoscintigraphy for detecting gastrointestinal and medullary thyroid cancers: first clinical results using radiolabeled monoclonal antibodies against carcinoembryonic antigen. Br Med J 1982; 285:1447–51.
8. Mach JP, Buchegger F, Forni M, et al. Use of radiolabeled monoclonal anti-CEA antibodies for the detection of human carcinomas by external photoscanning and tomoscintigraphy. Immunol Today 1981; 2:239–49.
9. Delaloye B, Bischof-Delaloye A, Buchegger F, et al. Detection of colorectal carcinoma by emission computerized tomography after injection of I-123 labeled Fab or F(ab')$_2$ fragments from monoclonal anti-carcinoembryonic antigen antibodies. J Clin Invest 1986; 77:301–11.
10. Abdel-Nabi HH, Schwartz AN, Higano CS, Wechter DG, Unger MW. Colorectal carcinoma: detection with indium-111 anticarcinoembryonic antigen monoclonal antibody ZCE 025. Radiology 1987; 164:617–21.
11. Abdel-Nabi HH, Schwartz AN, Goldfogel G, et al. Colorectal tumors; scintigraphy with In-111 anti-CEA monoclonal antibody and correlation with surgical, histopathologic, and immunohistochemical findings. Radiology 1988; 166:747–52.
12. Carrasquillo JA, Sugarbaker P, Colcher D, et al. Radioimmunoscintigraphy of colon cancer with iodine-131 labeled B72.3 monoclonal antibody. J Nucl Med 1988; 29:1022–30.
13. Yokoyama K, Carrasquillo JA, Chang AE, et al. Differences in biodistribution of indium-111 and iodine-131 labeled B72.3 monoclonal antibodies in patients with colorectal cancer. J Nucl Med 1989; 30:320–7.
14. Patt YZ, Lamki LM, Haynie TM, et al. Improved tumor localization with increasing dose of indium-111 labeled anticarcinoembryonic antigen monoclonal antibody ZCE 025 in metastatic colorectal cancer. J Clin Oncol 1988; 6:1220–30.
15. Lamki LM, Murray JL, Rosenblum MG, Patt YZ, Babaian R, Unger MW. Effect of unlabeled monoclonal antibody (MoAb) on biodistribution of 111 indium labeled (MoAb). Nucl Med Commun 1988; 9:553–64.
16. Halpern SE, Haindl W, Beauregard J, Hagan P, Clutter M, Amox D, Merchant B, Unger M, Mongovi C, Bartholomew R, Jue R, Carlo D, Dillman R.

Scintigraphy with In-111 labeled monoclonal antitumor antibodies: kinetics, biodistribution and tumor detection. Radiology 1988; 168:529–36.

17. Maguire RT, Schmelter RF, Pascussi VL, Conklin JJ. Immunoscintigraphy of colorectal adenocarcinoma: results with site-specifically radiolabeled B72.3 (^{111}In-CYT-103). Antibody Immunoconjugates, Radiopharm 1989; 2:257–69.

18. Abdel-Nabi H, Doerr R, Roth SC, Farrell E, Schmelter R, Maguire R. Biodistribution and tumor localization following varying doses of CYT-103 monoclonal antibody labeled with In-111 in colorectal carcinoma patients. J Nucl Med 1989; 767–8.

19. Abdel-Nabi H, Doerr RJ, Chan HW, Balu D, Schmelter RF, Maguire RT. In-111-labeled monoclonal antibody immunoscintigraphy in colorectal carcinoma: safety, sensitivity, and preliminary clinical results. Radiology 1990; 175:163–71.

20. Hsu SM, Raine L, Fanger H. Use of the avidin-biotin peroxidase complex (ABC) in immunoperoxidase techniques: a comparison between ABC and unlabeled (PAP) procedures. J Histochem Cytochem 1981; 29:577–80.

21. Hsu SM, Soban E. Color modifications of the diaminobenzadine (DAB) precipitation by metallic ions and its application for double immunohistochemistry. J Histochem Cytochem 1982; 30:1079–82.

22. Beatty JD, Hyams DM, Morton BA, Beatty BG, Williams LE, Yamauchi D, Merchant B, Paxton RJ, Shively JE. Impact of radiolabeled antibody imaging on management of colon cancer. Am J Surg 1989; 157:13–9.

23. Herrera L, Nabi H, Petrelli N, Vial G, Madrid R. Imaging with In-111 labeled anti-TAG (tumor associated glycoprotein) monoclonal antibody B72.3 (CYT-103) in patients with advanced colorectal cancer. Proceedings of the 15th International Cancer Congress, Hamburg, W. Germany, August, 1990.

24. Beahrs OH, Higgins GA, Weinstein JJ. In: Colorectal tumors. Philadelphia: Lippincott, 1986:141–313.

25. Wanebo HJ, Rao B, Pinsky CM, et al. The use of the preoperative carcinoembryonic antigen level as a prognostic indicator to complement pathologic staging. N Engl J Med 1978; 299:448.

26. Wanebo HJ, Stearns M, Schwartz MK. Use of CEA as an indicator of early recurrence and as a guide to a selected second look procedure in patients with colorectal cancer. Ann Surg 1978; 188:481.

27. Moertel CG, Shutt AJ, Go ULV. Carcinoembryonic antigen test for recurrent colorectal cancer. Inadequacy for early detection. JAMA 1978; 239:1065–6.

28. Sardi A, Minton JP, Nieroda C, Sickle-Santanello B, Young D, Martin EW, Jr. Multiple reoperations in recurrent colorectal carcinoma. An analysis of morbidity, mortality and survival. Cancer 1988; 61:1913–9.

29. Adson MA, Van Heerden JA, Adson MH, Wagner JS, Ilstrup DM. Resection of hepatic metastases from colorectal cancer. Arch Surg 1984; 119:647–51.

30. Horan Hand P, Colcher D, Salomen D, Ridge J, Noguchi P, Schlom J. Influence of spatial configuration of carcinoma cell populations on the expression of a tumor associated glycoprotein. Cancer Res 1985; 45:833–40.

31. Pacella M, Roth S, Gona J, Abdel-Nabi H. Determination of optimum imaging time of colorectal carcinoma patients infused with In-111 CYT-103 monoclonal antibodies. J Nucl Med Technol 1989; 17:113.

32. Sugarbaker PM, Gianola FJ, Dwyer A, et al. A simplified plan for follow-up of patients with colon and rectal cancer supported by prospective studies of laparotomy and radiologic test results. Surgery 1987; 102:79–87.
33. Moss AA. Imaging of colorectal carcinoma. Radiology 1989; 170:308–10.
34. Doerr RJ, Abdel-Nabi H, Merchant B. Indium-111 ZCE 025 immunoscintigraphy in occult recurrent colorectal cancer with elevated carcinoembryonic antigen level. Arch Surg 1990; 125:226–9.

6

Oncoscint CR103 Imaging in the Surgical Management of Patients with Colorectal Cancer

Ralph J. Doerr and Hani H. Abdel-Nabi
State University of New York at Buffalo, Buffalo, New York

INTRODUCTION

Colorectal carcinoma remains one of the main causes of death from cancer for both sexes. There appears to have been a slight increase in the incidence of colon cancer in the past 20 years [1]. Surgery remains the mainstay of treatment for primary and recurrent disease, with the 5-year survival (all stages) following curative resection of a primary colorectal cancer being about 40%. Approximately 25% of the patients will present with extensive, probably incurable, disease at initial diagnosis [2]. That 50% of patients with colorectal cancer have occult micrometastatic disease at the time of presentation bespeaks the need for more accurate preoperative staging. Currently, determination of the extent of disease at initial presentation entails performance of colonoscopy and/or barium enema, liver function tests, serum carcinoembryonic antigen (CEA) measurement, liver/spleen scan, and ultrasound or computed tomographic (CT) scan. The role of magnetic resonance imaging (MRI) as a preoperative tool has yet to be defined. A new addition to this diagnostic armamentarium is immunoscintigraphy using radiolabeled monoclonal antibodies.

Recently, several monoclonal antibodies to CEA or tumor-associated glycoprotein TAG-72, which is present on approximately 80% of adenocarcinomas, have been successfully labeled with radionuclides and investigated for the imaging of colorectal carcinoma in humans [3]. In these studies, excellent tumor localization has been achieved, and no major toxicities have been reported [4]. Primary tumors, as well as recurrent and metastatic lesions, have been imaged with a sensitivity of 70–85%, and a specificity consistently greater than 90% has been achieved [5]. In this chapter, we will define the role of this new technique in preoperative staging and postoperative follow-up and describe the potential impact of the procedure on clinical decision making and patient management.

CURRENT STAGING TECHNIQUES
Presurgical Staging of Colorectal Cancer
Colonoscopy

Significant advances in endoscopic visualization of the colon and anorectum have been made in the past 20 years. Data from rigid sigmoidoscopy have been supplemented by the use of the 60-cm flexible sigmoidoscope. Finally, total colonoscopy to the cecum has unquestionably led to discovery of polyps and cancers at earlier stages. When total colonoscopy is performed in newly detected colorectal cancer, synchronous carcinomas are found in 3–4% and additional benign polyps in 12% of patients [6].

In patients who cannot tolerate colonoscopy, double-contrast barium enema may be used as a substitute. However, 10% of neoplastic lesions detectable by colonoscopy will be missed by double-contrast barium enema [7]. An additional alternative involves the combined use of 60-cm sigmoidoscopy and double-contrast barium enema.

The optimal use of total colonoscopy, flexible sigmoidoscopy, and double-contrast barium enema, either alone or in combination, has not been definitively established. Total colonoscopy is appreciably more expensive than double-contrast barium enema and is associated with a significantly higher perforation rate [8]. The advantages of biopsy of the primary lesion and additonal lesion detection with colonoscopy must be seriously considered.

Barium Enema

In the 80 years that the colon has been examined by x-ray with contrast agents, significant refinements of the procedure have been made. Solid colon examinations have given way to air-insufflated, double-contrast barium enemas. Although the latter technique is a clear improvement for the detection of colon cancer, the error rate lies somewhere between 8.4 and 20% [9,10]. For small, colonic polyps (<1 cm), the bowel prep must be excellent. Patient cooperation and the radiologist's interpretation must similarly be superb. Barium enema is particularly helpful for surveillance of the lumen after colostomy. The lack of a seal around the stoma makes colonoscopy very difficult in this circumstance. The complication rate, particularly perforation, is under 1%

[11]. Cardiac arrhythmias can be induced with the insufflation necessary for an adequate examination. Generally, however, barium enema is quite well tolerated even by elderly patients.

Perhaps the optimal diagnostic approach for detection of disease in the colonic lumen is the combination of endoscopy and air contrast barium enema. An error rate of only 3% for right-sided lesions was reported when these two modalities were combined [7]. Colonoscopy and barium enema are complementary procedures in the diagnosis of colonic malignancy.

CEA

Since its discovery in 1965, CEA has become the standard serum tumor-associated antigen to follow in the management of colorectal cancer patients [12]. Unfortunately, the CEA assay has failed as a pure screening or diagnostic test because of a high false positive rate in cigarette smokers and patients with chronic lung and liver disease [13]. Elevations detected in a series of other solid-organ carcinomas (breast, ovary) further diminish its value for differential diagnosis [14].

The benefit of the CEA assay is more obvious when the assay results are considered in relation to the stage of colorectal cancer. The rate of assay positivity correlates with the Dukes staging classification [15]. While elevated CEA levels can be detected in only 25% of Dukes' A lesions, 61% of Dukes' C tumors are associated with elevated CEA in the peripheral blood. When distant metastatic disease is present, 86% of the patients have an elevated CEA [16].

Poorly differentiated and heavy mucin-producing carcinomas do not express CEA in the serum to the same degree as moderately differentiated lesions. There is some correlation with level of CEA and ultimate survival, such that preoperative CEA levels greater than 20 ng/mL are predictive of future local recurrence or distant metastases [17].

The greatest utility of this assay is in detecting recurrent colorectal cancer. It is critical to obtain the first baseline CEA level prior to the initial surgical procedure. The CEA test should then be performed every 4 months for the next 2 years, the period during which 70% of the recurrences develop [17]. An elevation in CEA should prompt a second serum determination to verify the result. Confirmed elevations should dictate an aggressive diagnostic workup to identify potentially resectable recurrences. It is possible to determine the slope of the increase in CEA and make a relative prediction of the site of the recurrence. A slow rise in CEA signifies a local or regional recurrence, while a steep rise more likely represents a parenchymal metastasis, usually in the liver [18].

The choice of the appropriate clinical path to follow after identifying a postoperative rise in CEA remains in question. Certainly an elevated CEA level will prompt a search for recurrence. Whether CEA-directed and second-look procedures that result in tumor resection increase overall survival is under study at present [19]. Finally, another use for serial CEA examinations is the follow-up of patients receiving chemotherapy and radiotherapy. A positive response, indicated by a significant decrease from the elevated pretreatment CEA level, corresponds to a longer disease-free interval and a higher survival rate [20].

Ultrasound

The extremely important task of accurately staging the extent of colorectal cancer has been appreciably advanced by ultrasound. The patterns of local-regional spread and metastatic disease are well described [21]. With the present technology, it is possible to detect 1- to 2-cm lesions, and in some circumstances, lesions less than 1 cm [22].

In the liver, ultrasound has demonstrated consistently high sensitivities, detecting approximately 85% of hepatic metastases [23]. Specificity reaches 82% in some series. The examination can be safely and quickly repeated as often as necessary without causing discomfort to the patient.

In the liver, the differential diagnosis of an ultrasound-detected lesion includes hematoma, abscess, cyst, or tumor. Each of these disease processes has specific ultrasound criteria for diagnosis [24]. One area of difficulty arises with the regenerating nodule in a cirrhotic liver [24]. Also, it may be quite difficult to differentiate a primary liver tumor from metastatic disease. The "bull's eye" configuration of a metastatic nodule has been well described [25]. The advantage of being able to perform ultrasound-guided needle biopsy has also expanded the role of this modality in differential diagnosis and staging.

Ultrasound has had varying success in the detection of lymph node metastases [26]. Regional lymph node metastases ordinarily must achieve a size of 2 cm before they can be distinguished from normal lymph nodes [27]. While the specificity exceeds 90%, the false negative rate can exceed 50% [28]. The inability to detect half the nodes containing disease impairs the accuracy and predictability of the test.

More extensive colorectal cancer may present with involvement of contiguous organs or the abdominal cavity itself. Ultrasound has been recognized as being unparalleled for detecting free ascites and loculated fluid in the peritoneal cavity [29]. Tumor extending locally beyond the confines of the bowel is not as accurately described with this modality. If the lesion is in a sonographically favorable position, it is possible to perform fine-needle aspiration biopsy.

Considering the relative ease of obtaining and performing the examination, ultrasound becomes a reasonable test to begin the workup for local and metastatic spread of colorectal cancer. Should the ultrasound findings prove equivocal, or if technical difficulties supervene (open wound, stoma, gas distention, obesity), other modalities − CT, MRI and monoclonal antibody (MAb) scanning − must be used sooner.

CT/MRI

The advantages of CT scan in the detection of early metastases and recurrences have been well documented. In the liver, the CT scan provides an accuracy unparalleled by any other cross-sectional imaging modality. The sensitivity and specificity for hepatic metastases approach 90% [30]. The size of the metastatic deposit routinely imaged depends on the cuts through the liver, but 1-cm lesions can be reproducibly detected [31]. Even smaller lesions were found with lipoid contrast, EOE-13 enhancement, before this agent was removed from the market [32]. Identification of a metastatic nodule in the liver can lead to stereotactic-guided needle biopsy.

MRI provides a complementary role to CT scanning for tumor detection in the liver. While data are limited, hepatic lesions as small as 0.5 cm have been identified [33]. More importantly, MRI beautifully demonstrates the parenchymal vasculature, thus permitting consideration of nodule relationship to critical hepatic and portal vessels. This aspect is advantageous in designing a potential operation to deal safely and definitively with metastatic disease in the liver.

Areas in which we have found the CT scan to be deficient preoperatively are: detection of depth of tumor wall penetration, including adjacent organ involvement, and detection of lymph node and pelvic recurrences [34]. As local recurrence is a particularly difficult problem with rectal cancer, the need for an imaging tool to obviate the difficulties encountered by CT scan regarding differentiation of postoperative changes from residual/recurrent disease becomes apparent. Although MRI has shown superiority to CT in some series, difficulty with radiation changes in the pelvis reduces this modality's efficacy [35]. As more rectal cancers are adjuvantly managed with radiotherapy pre- and postoperatively, interpretative problems due to radiation changes will become more common.

The immunoscintigraphic and cross-sectional imaging modalities should be thought of as complementary. Even with the increased accuracy, there remain anatomical areas difficult to image. The diaphragm, root of mesentery, pelvis, nodal metastases, local extent of tumor, small synchronous lesions, regional postoperative changes, and other benign disease entities are among the challenges for these diagnostic tools. It is in these areas that radiolabeled monoclonal antibody imaging will find its greatest utility and contribute significantly to patient management.

Clinicopathological Staging of Colorectal Cancer
Tumor Characteristics

Once the diagnosis of carcinoma of the colon or rectum has been established, the treatment offered to the patient will be profoundly affected by the preoperative staging. The ultimate prognosis will depend on the pathological examination of the resected specimen. A number of features of the tumor appear to influence the patient's prognosis. The following specific characteristics of the tumor itself have prognostic importance: size of tumor (greater or less than 2 cm); site of primary tumor (colon has better prognosis overall than rectum); type (sessile and ulcerated are worse than polypoid); presence of complete bowel obstruction or perforation; extent of infiltration through bowel wall (closer to serosa worsens survival); differentiation of tumor; and presence of cytological features (signet-ring, mucinous changes as well as flow cytometric characteristics, e.g., diploid versus aneuploid and mitotic indices) all have predictive value in determining the 5-year survival of the patient (36).

The most important determinant in survival is the documentation of lymph node metastases [37]. The site of the lymph node involvement (the more distant from the bowel wall, the more dismal the prognosis) and the number of involved lymph nodes (no nodal involvement versus one to four nodes versus more than four nodes) are critical to prognosis. Also, the presence or absence of venous or perineural involvement indicates the aggressiveness of the tumor and correlates with the potential for distal spread [38].

There is some evidence that host immunological response is related to survival [39]. Patients who seem to elicit a strong inflammatory response, particularly around the tumor itself and in the lymph nodes, appear to have a better prognosis.

Dukes' Staging

The mainstay of clinical decision making remains the Dukes classification. As described by Dukes in 1932, the two most important findings are whether the tumor has penetrated the muscularis mucosa and whether the lymph nodes are involved with tumor [40]. Originally, Dukes' A referred to tumors that had not reached the muscularis mucosa and demonstrated no lymph node metastases. Dukes' B classified a tumor that extended to or through the serosa but remained without evidence of lymph node metastases. Finally, Dukes' C defined a tumor of any depth with lymph node metastases. There have been numerous attempts to refine the Dukes classification. The modification we have found most useful is that of Gunderson and Sosin, who, in 1974, established $B_{1,2,3}$ and $C_{1,2,3}$ categories in which invaded adjacent organs were classified as B_3 and adjacent organ involvement with lymph node metastases was designated C_3 [41]. Further subdivision to categorize gross involvement (g) and microscopic involvement (m) has helped to better determine extent. The final useful addition came from the Gastrointestinal Tumor Study Group (1975), who stratified their patients with lymph node metastases into those with four or fewer involved lymph nodes (C_1) or those with five or more involved lymph nodes (C_2) [42].

The ultimate value of any staging scheme is its ability to establish 5- and 10-year survival rates. The Astler-Collier modification of the Dukes classification found the following 5-year survivals: stage A = 100%, B = 66.6%; B_2 = 53.9%; C_1 = 42.8%; C_2 = 22.4% [43]. These rates can be further refined for individual patients by taking into account clinical symptoms (the asymptomatic patient fares much better) as well as the intrinsic characteristics of the tumor outlined above. One additional, extremely important aspect of this classification system is the ability to predict which patients will have recurrence and what pattern (local-regional versus distant) the recurrence will take.

IMMUNOSCINTIGRAPHY
MAb Imaging of Primary Colorectal Cancer

Of the 165,000 patients presenting yearly with colorectal carcinoma, only 40% will be alive 5 years after the diagnosis [1]. Methods that could detect more extensive or occult disease at initial presentation may impact beneficially on this survival figure.

Surgery remains the mainstay of therapy for this disease. Although the incidence of colorectal carcinoma has increased over the past several decades, the distribution of localized versus disseminated disease does not appear to have changed [1]. If the in situ cancers and cancerous polyps are excluded, the overall survival rates remain essentially unchanged since the 1950s. Despite the dramatic changes in early detection (endoscopy, Hemoccult R), stool examination, air contrast barium enema, and the use of more effective surgical procedures (the profound decrease in abdominal-perineal resections and concomitant rise in anterior resections, concepts of en bloc cancer resection, wide lymphadenectomy, synchronous solid-organ metastases resection, adjuvant pre- and postoperative radiation, and newer chemotherapeutic regimens), cures still occur in only half the patients.

Staging at the time of presentation is clearly linked to the ultimate prognosis for the patient. At present, staging of colorectal cancer is incomplete, being limited by surgical and pathological classifications. It is felt that individual patient management would be profoundly benefitted by more accurate staging.

To this end, once the diagnosis of a primary lesion has been established by barium enema or colonoscopy, a number of newer diagnostic imaging modalities have been employed to attempt to refine the stage, affect management, and, finally, increase survival.

The newest addition to the presurgical examination for staging of primary colorectal cancer is the radiolabeled MAb directed against tumor-associated antigens. One such MAb, B72.3, has been extensively investigated as a tumor-imaging agent to identify the anatomical distribution of malignancy using immunoscintigraphy [3]. In initial studies, ^{131}I-B72.3 localized to 70% of tumor lesions with very favorable tumor-tissue background ratios [4]. In further work, when given intraperitoneally, the radiolabeled MAb detected tumor lesions missed by conventional diagnostic tests in 25% of patients [44]. Since probably 50% of patients presenting with colorectal cancer harbor heretofore occult micrometastatic disease, the role of this modality in preoperative staging begins to be crystallized.

In a large multicenter trial involving 103 patients, including 61 evaluated for primary disease, B72.3-GYK-DTPA (CYT-103) radiolabeled with ^{111}In correctly identified colorectal adenocarcinoma lesions with a 70% sensitivity [45]. Importantly, the antibody scan was negative in 9 of 10 patients who were free of malignancy (90% specificity). In 5 of 55 patients with surgically confirmed primary colorectal cancer, ^{111}In-CYT-103 immunoscintigraphy detected occult lesions. More extensive regional or metastatic disease, including bone metastasis, carcinomatosis, and nodal disease, was detected. Also, another primary lesion not detected at the presurgical workup was discovered by the MAb scan.

Critical to the perspective of imaging in colorectal cancer is the impact that radiolabeled MAb scintigraphy has had on patient management. Increased knowledge of the extent and spread of tumor has significant implications for therapy. Figure 1 is an anterior planar MAb scan of a 66-year-old man with a right colon primary cancer and left supraclavicular lymphadenopathy (Virchow's node). The initial pathology report from a biopsy of the supraclavicular lymph nodes revealed disease consistent with squamous cell carcinoma. The final pathology report revealed metastatic adenocarcinoma consistent with the right colon primary. Disregard of immunoscintigraphic findings in this case would have led to unnecessary major head and neck surgery.

In the primary setting, an antibody scan showing extensive local and regional spread suggests benefits may be derived by preoperative or intraoperative radiotherapy. The demonstration that there is no distant intra-abdominal or extra-abdominal spread in the patient would support an aggressive regimen of preoperative radiation in an attempt to convert a lesion from inoperable to operable. Figure 2 is a MAb scan that reveals a massive rectal tumor but no other evidence of spread. These findings supported an aggressive

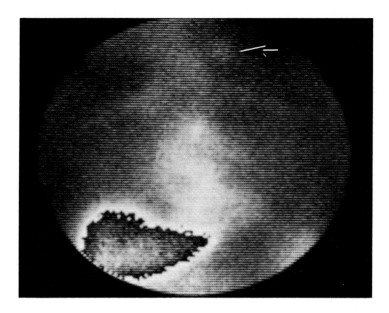

Figure 1 Anterior planar thoracic image of a patient with primary colon cancer and left supraclavicular lymphadenopathy (arrow).

preoperative radiotherapy course followed by pelvic exenterative surgery. No extrapelvic tumor was found at operation, confirming the scan findings.

Extensive local tumor or regional lymph node metastases bolster the concept of wider margins of resection and extended lymphadenectomies. Rosemurgy et al. reported markedly improved 5- and 10-year survival rates (78.1 and 60.9%, respectively) for colon cancer patients managed with wide, en bloc anatomical resection and extensive lymph node dissection [46].

MAb scans demonstrating synchronous colon lesions argue for extended hemicolectomy or subtotal colectomy. Another subset of patients who potentially may benefit from immunoscintigraphy are those with small, dysplastic colonic lesions, ulcerative colitis, or familial polyposis. The patient with ulcerative colitis for more than 5 years or dysplasia on routine biopsy would be an excellent candidate for MAb scanning to search for possible invasive carcinoma and, therefore, help define the need for earlier colectomy.

Twenty-five percent of patients presenting with colorectal cancer already have hepatic metastases [2]. Preoperative knowledge of these metastases by MAb scan would alter the operative approach by suggesting a more extensive workup, including celiac axis, SMA, hepatic artery angiography, and liver MRI to determine the extent and resectability of these hepatic deposits and/or to make decisions regarding implantation of a hepatic artery chemotherapeutic device.

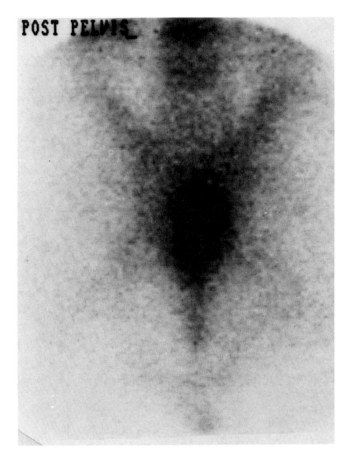

Figure 2 Posterior pelvic CYT-103 image demonstrating a large rectal tumor.

Critical to decision making in the preoperative evaluation of the primary lesion is the determination of extra-abdominal spread. Beatty et al. reported the major impact of MAb scanning to be in the detection of extra-abdominal metastases [47]. Further investigations of these lesions, including fine-needle aspiration biopsy, permitted initiation of radiation and chemotherapeutic treatments that often obviated the need for a surgical procedure.

While the role of immunoscintigraphy in the preoperative phase of a primary colorectal carcinoma is still being defined, there are ample data to support its continued use with the expectation of significant impact on clinical decision making [48]. Table 1 describes our regimen for more accurate preoperative staging of primary colorectal cancer.

Table 1 Preoperative Staging of Primary
Colorectal Carcinoma

Full colonoscopy/air-contrast barium enema
Chest x-ray
Carcinoembryonic antigen and liver function tests
Intravenous pyelogram
Computerized tomography scan
Monoclonal antibody scan

MAb Imaging of Recurrent/Metastatic Colorectal Cancer

Surveillance Strategy: Follow-up Imaging Protocol for Patients at Risk

Surgical resection of primary colorectal cancer cures only 50% of patients. The remaining 50% will die of locally recurrent and/or metastatic disease within 5 years of the intial presentation [2]. The great preponderance of recurrences occur within the first 2 postoperative years [17]. Half the recurrences are asymptomatic, and if one waits until symptoms become evident, chances for a meaningful surgical intervention are markedly lessened. Programs of intensified follow-up have seemingly failed in the past owing to low reresection rates and poor long-term survival in patients subjected to curative reoperation. If the recurrences and metastases can be identified sooner and more accurately, the opportunity for a good clinical outcome is enhanced. Local recurrence is found in 40% of patients following curative resection for primary colorectal cancer [17]. Five-year survival rates of up to 26% have recently been reported in the absence of distant metastases if reresection is done early [49].

First, one must identify patients at highest risk for recurrence. Clearly, when the tumor has penetrated the bowel wall (Dukes' B_2), is adherent to or has invaded adjacent organs (Dukes' B_3), or contains lymph node metastases (Dukes' C_{2-3}), the chance for recurrence is increased. The timing and intensity of surveillance must be directed to those at greatest risk in the critical first 2 years after primary resection.

The type and sequence of follow-up examinations to employ are in question. Many different regimens have been suggested and have cheifly involved periodic clinical examination, colonoscopy and/or air contrast barium enema, chest x-ray, serial blood counts, chemistries, and serum CEA determinations. Identification of any possible abnormality or persistent symptoms routinely leads to cross-sectional imaging, i.e., ultrasound (US), CT, or MRI. Within this context, the addition of immunoscintigraphy directed toward patients with Dukes' B_2 and higher stages in the first 2 years postoperatively can be anticipated

Table 2 Follow-up Protocol in High-Risk Colorectal Cancer Patients (Dukes' B_2 or greater)

Regular visits	Every 4 months x 2 years; then every 6 mos x 3 years
Monoclonal antibody scan	Every 6 mos x 2 years; then yearly x 3 years
Liver function tests and carcinoembryonic antigen	With each office visit
Colonoscopy	Yearly, alternating with air-contrast barium enema
Chest x-ray	Yearly
Computerized tomography/ bone/brain scans	Dictated by signs and symptoms

to have its greatest impact. Table 2 is the recommended follow-up regimen for patients with Dukes B_2 lesions or higher stages.

Utilized at regular 6-month intervals in this high-risk group, immunoscintigraphy can be expected to identify recurrence or metastases at a much earlier and more favorable stage. By working in concert with the other imaging and serum diagnostic modalities and complementing their unique advantages, significant palliation, better prognostication, and ultimately improved survival can be anticipated with the addition of MAb scanning. In the multicenter trial mentioned previously, ^{111}In-CYT-103 imaging detected surgically confirmed recurrences in 24 of 37 patients (65%). This included the detection of previously occult lesions in six patients, including two patients with elevated CEA levels and otherwise negative diagnostic workups. Importantly, antibody scans were negative in four of four patients with no evidence of disease at second-look surgery (100% specificity). In the following sections, the potential impact of antibody imaging will be described for various subsets of patients with recurrent disease.

Abdominal and Pelvic Recurrence

Endoscopy is unparalleled in the diagnosis of intraluminal recurrence, finding approximately 94% of these lesions [50]. Immunoscintigraphy, because of its high specificity, has its greatest impact on extraluminal recurrence.

Postoperative changes render interpretation of conventional cross-sectional imaging (CT, US, MRI) exceedingly difficult. As tumor antigen expression generally is independent of serum CEA or TAG-72 elevations, the evaluation of new symptoms, e.g., pelvic pain, by MAb imaging should not be withheld in patients with normal serum levels of these assays.

While early detection and aggressive surgery have been controversial, recent findings have tempered the original pessimism concerning operations for recurrent lesions. An Austrian group reporting on surgery for local recurrences found that 87% of patients with recurrence were able to undergo an operation [51]. Half the operations were felt to be radical and curative in intent. The remaining 50% were palliative. Of patients who underwent reoperations for potential cure, 30% survived 35 months or more. A second local recurrence after radical surgery was seen in 28% and, again, was manageable surgically. The palliative group was significantly helped by confirmation of diagnosis and the institution of radiation and chemotherapy. Relief of obstruction and bleeding, as well as control of pain, was established in over 80% of the cases. The investigators' conclusion that 5-year survival rates of 33% may be obtained after surgery for local recurrence is predicated on the detection of recurrent disease at an early stage and, therefore, further supports the present thesis.

The addition of intraoperative radiotherapy to the local regional resective bed has also preliminarily proved useful.

Hepatic Metastasis

At present, the patients who stand the best chance of deriving long-term survival benefit from reoperative resection procedures are those with metastatic disease confined to the liver. Figure 3 is a MAb scan that demonstrates isolated liver metastasis 1 year following resection of a sigmoid colon tumor. No other evidence of disease was confirmed at the time of hepatic resection.

Multiple series have demonstrated a 20–25% 5-year survival rate after resection of colorectal cancer metastatic to the liver [52–54]. The Pittsburgh group reports 5-year survivals of 40% in this subset of patients [55].

Preoperative staging in this group is critical because the presence of extrahepatic metastases is an absolute contraindication to liver resection [56]. Interestingly, multiple liver metastases, provided they are accessible to removal, do not diminish the survival benefit of resection. While Dukes' B primary lesions appear to fare better than Dukes' C when metastatic to the liver, other factors such as synchronous versus metachronous lesions and size and location of metastases do not provide additonal prognostic information [52]. There does seem to be an improved survival benefit when metastases appear 2 years or more after primary resection, which may reflect intrinsic tumor biology and host defense factors [53].

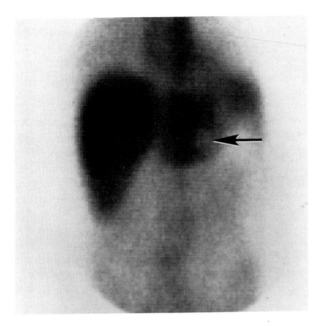

Figure 3 Isolated hepatic metastasis (arrow) 1 year after primary colon cancer resection.

Distant Metastasis: Lung, Bone

Chest radiographs and CT scanning are unsurpassed in detecting lung and mediastinal metastases. These techniques, although sensitive, lack specificity. Figure 4 is a MAb scan demonstrating a lung metastasis in a patient with a known pelvic recurrence. The confirmation of lung metastasis contributed to cancellation of the proposed pelvic tumor resection and institution of appropriate therapy. Immunoscintigraphy can assist CT scan in the differentiation of benign and malignant lung parenchymal lesions and mediastinal adenopathy <1.5 cm.

While radionuclide bone scanning is the most sensitive examination for identifying bone metastases, there is a complementary role for immunoscintigraphy. Figure 5 shows MAb scans in a patient following abdominal perineal resection for rectal cancer. The MAb scan was the initial modality to detect bony metastases in the right shoulder, left sixth rib, and thoracic spine. These lesions were confirmed on bone scan. Furthermore, the left sixth rib lesion (demonstrated by both techniques) was biopsied and found to be metastatic. One drawback of ^{111}In-labeled antibodies is the increased bone marrow activity of the isotope, which could diminish its sensitivity for bony lesions. Despite

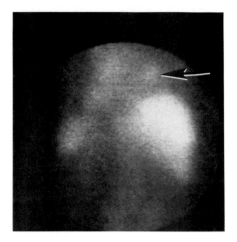

Figure 4 Posterior planar CYT-103 image demonstrating metastatic lung lesion (arrow) in patient with known pelvic recurrence.

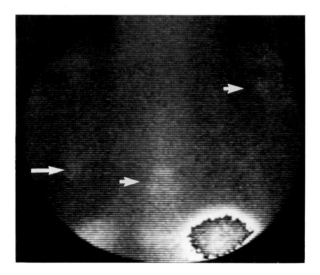

Figure 5 Posterior planar CYT-103 image demonstrating metastases to bone in right shoulder, left sixth rib, and thoracic spine (arrows).

this, the advantage of the MAb scan's specificity can be seen, particularly when a bony metastasis may mitigate against an exenterative pelvic procedure for recurrence or hepatic metastasis resection.

Occult Disease

The MAb scan appears to have a defined role in the preoperative workup of primary and recurrent colorectal cancer via its ability to detect tumor deposits in the lymph nodes and other soft tissues in the abdomen and retroperitoneal area that are commonly missed by currently available tests. The unique advantage of finding disease when all other examinations, including CEA, are negative is particularly appealing. Figure 6 is an example of a positive MAb scan in the face of a negative CT scan and physical examination in a patient without an elevated CEA level. The identification of occult disease in patients scheduled for second-look laparotomy for suspected recurrence helps define

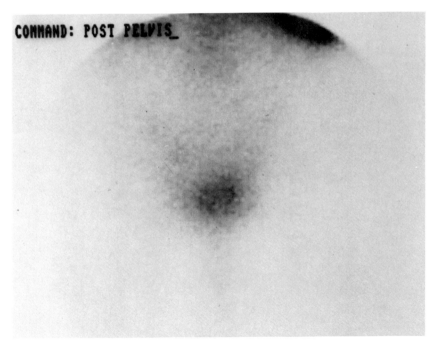

Figure 6 Pelvic tumor recurrence in patient without evidence of disease on physical examination or CT scan.

Table 3 Investigators' Assessment of the Impact of Antibody (MAb) Imaging on Patient Management

Effect of the MAb scan findings on management of the patient	Number of patients	(%)
Very beneficial	6/69	(9)
Beneficial	12/69	(17)
No effect	49/69	(71)
Negative	1/69	(1)
Very negative	1/69	(1)

the surgical procedure to be undertaken. This is of special benefit to patients with presumed isolated, resectable disease and patients with elevated serum CEA levels and negative conventional presurgical workup.

Patient Management

Within the context of patient management, the impact of antibody imaging has been assessed in a large subset of patients. Investigators utilizing ^{111}In-labeled CYT-103 as a presurgical diagnostic/staging modality considered immunoscintigraphy to be beneficial or very beneficial in 26% of patients [45] (Table 3). Advantages of the MAb scan included detection of previously occult lesions, identification of localized disease without regional or metastatic spread, and confirmation of adenocarcinoma when other diagnostic tests were equivocal. The ability to aid in the exclusion of recurrent or metastatic cancer when symptoms or conventional examinations are preliminarily positive is another important aspect of immunoscintigraphy.

Baum et al., reporting on a large patient experience, found immunoscintigraphy to be helpful, primarily in complementing other diagnostic methods, in 46% of patients [3]. In 20% of the cases, the MAb scan contributed unique information, identifying abdominal or lymph node metastases or pelvic recurrences missed by conventional workup. Finally, immunoscintigraphy was felt to contribute to a change in treatment strategy, e.g., institution of radiotherapy or second-look laparotomy, in 13% of patients.

CONCLUSION

The impact of colorectal cancer immunoscintigraphy on surgical decision making will alter the operative approach in approximately 25% of cases. The ability to more accurately define the presence and extent of tumor in primary patients will certainly contribute to their operative management. The ability to more accurately detect the extent of disease in patients with presumably localized, resectable, recurrent, or metastatic lesions and the ability to negate the surgical option when unresectable abdominal or extra-abdominal disease is found further defined the niche for this imaging modality. Thus, MAb scanning will contribute to the management of both primary- and recurrent-disease patients.

When compared to CT scanning, immunoscintigraphy correctly identified tumor lesions in patients with negative CT scans, while CT scanning found tumors in patients with negative MAb scans. CT is better in detecting hepatic lesions, while immunoscintigraphy identifies extrahepatic disease, including extra-abdominal lesions and those in the mid-abdomen and pelvis.

As a complementary tool to presurgical evaluation of the patient with primary, recurrent, and occult colorectal cancer, MAb scanning has shown that it can beneficially influence patient management.

REFERENCES

1. Cancer statistics. CA 1983; 33(1):2–25.
2. Wood DA, Robbins GF, Zobbin C, et al. Staging of cancer of the colon and rectum. Cancer 1979; 43:961–6.
3. Thor A, Ohuchi N, Szpak CA, Johnston WW, Schlom J. Distribution of oncofetal antigen TAG-72 defined by monoclonal antibody B72.3. Cancer Res 1986; 46:3118–24.
4. Carrasquillo JA, Sugarbaker P, Colcher D, et al. Radioimmunoscintigraphy of colon cancer with iodine-131 labeled B72.3 monoclonal antibody. J Nucl Med 1988; 29:1022–30.
5. Abdel-Nabi HH, Schwartz AN, Higano CS, Wechter DG, Unger MW. Colorectal carcinoma: detection with indium-111 anti-CEA monoclonal antibody ZCE-025. Radiology 1987; 164:617–21.
6. Miller SF, Knight AR. The early detection of colorectal cancer. Cancer 1977; 40:945.
7. Thoeni RF, Petras A. Double contrast barium enema and endoscopy in the detection of polypoid lesions in the cecum and ascending colon. Radiology 1982; 144:257.
8. Rogers BHG, Silvis SE, Nebel OF, et al. Complications of flexible colonoscopy and polypectomy. Gastrointest Endosc 1975; 22:73.
9. Ott DJ, Gelfand DW, Wu WC, Kerr RM. Sensitivity of double contrast barium enema: emphasis on polyp detection. Am J Roentgenol 1980; 135:327.
10. Kelvin FM, Gardiner R, Vas W, Stevenson GW. Colorectal carcinoma missed on double contrast barium enema study: a problem in perception. Am J Roentgenol 1981; 137:307.
11. Maglinte DDT, Strong RC, et al. Barium enema after colorectal biopsies. Experimental data. Am J Roentgenol 1982; 139:693.

12. Gold P, Freedman SO. Demonstration of tumor-specific antigens in human colon carcinoma by immunological tolerance absorption techniques. J Exp Med 1965; 121:439–62.

13. Martin EW Jr, Kibbey WE, DiVecchia L, et al. Carcinoembryonic antigen. Clinical and historic aspects. Cancer 1976; 37:62–81.

14. Mavligit GM, Stuckey S. Colorectal carcinoma. Evidence for circulating CEA-anti-CEA complexes. Cancer 1983; 52:146–9.

15. Midiori G, Amanti C, Consorti F, et al. Usefulness of preoperative CEA levels in the assessment of colorectal cancer patient stage. J Surg Oncol 1983; 22:257–60.

16. Evans JT, Mittelman A, Chu M, et al. Pre and postoperative uses of CEA. Cancer 1978; 42:1419–21.

17. Polk HC, Spratt JS Jr. Recurrent colorectal carcinoma: detection, treatment and other considerations. Surgery 1971; 69:9.

18. Staab HJ, Anderer FA, Stumpf E, et al. Slope analysis of the postoperative CEA time course and its possible application as an aid in diagnosis of disease progression in gastrointestinal cancer. Am J Surg 1978; 136:322–7.

19. Steele G Jr, Zamcheck N, Wilson R, et al. Results of CEA-initiated second-look surgery for recurrent colorectal cancer. Am J Surg 1980; 139:544–8.

20. Hine KR, Dykes PW. Prospective randomized trial of early cytotoxic therapy for recurrent colorectal carcinoma detected by serum CEA. Gut 1984; 25:682–8.

21. Gosgrove, DO. Clinic in diagnostic ultrasound. In: Goldberg BB, ed, Ultrasound in cancer. London:Churchill Livingston, 1981:1.

22. Bisker J, McCarthy J. Computerized tomographic demonstration of colonic carcinoma metastatic to the spleen. Comput Radiol 1983; 7(3):193–4.

23. Bartolozzi C, Ciarti S, Lucarelli E, et al. Ultrasound and computed tomography in the evaluation of focal liver disease. Acta Radiol Diagn 1981; 22(5):545.

24. Green B, Breen RL, Gostein HM, Stanley C. Gray-scale ultrasound evaluation of hepatic neoplasm: patterns and correlations. Radiology 1977; 124:203.

25. Scheible W, Gosink BB, Leopold GR. Gray-scale echographic patterns of hepatic metastatic disease. Am J Roentgenol 1977; 129:983.

26. Asher WM, Freimans AK. Echographic diagnosis of retroperitoneal lymph node enlargement. Ultrasound technique and diagnostic findings. Am J Roentgenol 1969; 105:438.

27. Subramanian BR, Balthazar EJ, Horri SCC, Hitton S. Abdominal lymphadenopathy in intravenous drug addicts: Sonographic features and clinical significance. Am J Roentgenol 1985; 144:917.

28. Pardes JG, Auh YH, Kneeland JB, et al. The oblique coronal view in sonography of the retroperitoneum. Am J Roentgenol 1985; 14:1241.

29. Bundrick TJ, Cho SR, Brewer WH, Beachler MC. Ascites: comparison of plain film radiographs with ultrasound. Radiology 1983; 148:875.

30. Levitt G, Sagel SS, Stanley RJ, Jost RG. Accuracy of computerized tomography of the liver and biliary tract. Radiology 1977; 124:123.

31. Heikem JP, Lee JKT, Glazer HS, Ling D. Hepatic metastasis studied with MR and CT. Radiology 1985; 156:423.

32. Miller DL, Vermess M, Doppman JC, et al. CT of the liver and spleen with EOE-13: review of 225 examinations. Am J Roentgenol 1984; 143:235.

33. Stark DD, Wittenberg J, Middleton MS, Ferrucci JT. Liver metastases: detection by phase contrast MR imaging. Radiology 1986; 158:327.

34. Freeny PC, Marks WM, Ryan JA, Bolen JW. Colorectal carcinoma evaluation with CT: preoperative staging and detection of postoperative recurrence. Radiology 1986; 158:347.

35. Glazer HS, Lee JKT, Levitt RG, et al. Radiation fibrosis: differentiation from recurrent tumor by MR imaging. Radiology 1985; 156:721.

36. Qizilbash AH. Pathologic studies in colorectal cancer: a guide to the surgical pathology examination of colorectal specimens and review of features of prognostic significance. In: Sommers SC, Rosen PP, eds.: Pathology annual. Part 1. Vol 17. Norwalk, CT:Appleton-Century-Crofts, 1982:1.

37. Osnes S. Carcinoma of the colon and rectum. A study of 353 cases with special reference to prognosis. Acta Chir Scand 1955; 110:378.

38. Talbot IC, Ritchie S, Leighton MH, et al. Spread of rectal cancer within veins: histologic features and clinical significance. Am J Surg 1981; 141:15.

39. Greco RS. Relation between immunity and survival in carcinoma of the colon and rectum. Am J Surg 1979; 137:752–6.

40. Dukes CE. The classification of cancer of the rectum. J Pathol Bacteriol 1932; 35:322–32.

41. Gunderson LL, Sosin H. Areas of failure found at reoperation following curative surgery for adenocarcinoma of the rectum. Clinicopathologic correlations and implications for adjuvant therapy. Cancer 1974; 34:1278.

42. Scheiu PS, et al. Adjuvant chemotherapy and radiotherapy following rectal surgery: an interim report of the Gastrointestinal Tumor Study Group (GITSG). In: James SE, Salmon SE, eds. Adjuvant therapy of cancer. Vol III. New York:Grune & Stratton. 1981:547.

43. Astler VB, Collier FA. The prognostic significance of direct extension of carcinoma of the colon and rectum. Ann Surg 1954; 139:846.

44. Carrasquillo JA, Sugarbaker P, Colcher D, et al. Peritoneal carcinomatosis imaging with intraperitoneal injection of I-131 labeled B72.3 monoclonal antibody. Radiology 1988; 167:35–40.

45. Doerr RJ, Abdel-Nabi H, Krag D, Mitchell E. Radiolabeled antibody imaging in the management of colorectal cancer: results of a multicenter clinical study. Ann Surg (in press).

46. Rosemurgy AS, Block GE, Shihab F. Surgical treatment of carcinoma of the abdominal colon. Surg Gynecol Obstet 1988; 167:399–406.

47. Beatty J, Hyams D, Morton B, et al. Impact of radiolabeled antibody imaging on management of colon cancer. Am J Surg 1989; 157:13–9.

48. Doerr RJ, Abdel-Nabi HH, Merchant B. In-111 ZCE-025 immunoscintigraphy in occult recurrent colorectal cancer with elevated CEA. Arch Surg 1990; 125:226–9.

49. Mentges B, Bruckner R. Das kolokarzinom: Prognostische faktoren. Dtsch Med Wochenschr 1986; 11:1790.

50. Welch JP, Donaldson GA. Detection and treatment of recurrent cancer of colon and rectum. Am J Surg 1978; 135:505.

51. Baum RP, Lorenz M, Hottenoot C, Staz-Sebler E, Hissnauer G, et al. The clinical application of immunoscintigraphy: results of a prospective study controlled by surgery, histology and immunohistochemistry and compared to CT-Scan and sonography. Nucl Med 1987; 26(4):35.

52. Butler J, Attiyeh FF, Daly JM. Hepatic resection for metastases of the colon and rectum. Surg Gynecol Obstet 1986; 162:109–13.

53. Adson MA, Van Heerden JA, Adson MH, et al. Resection of hepatic metastases from colorectal cancer. Arch Surg 1984; 119:647.

54. Cady B, McDermott WV. Major hepatic resection for metachronous metastases from colon cancer. Ann Surg 1985; 201:204–9.

55. Iwatsuki S, Shaw BW, Starzl TE. Experience with 150 liver resections. Ann Surg 1983; 197:247.

56. Hughes KS, Simon RM, Songhorabodi S, et al. Resection of the liver for colorectal carcinoma metastases: a multi-institutional study of indications for resection. Surgery 1988; 103:278–88.

7

Multicenter Clinical Trial of ^{111}In-CYT-103 in Patients with Ovarian Cancer

Donald G. Gallup

Medical College of Georgia, Augusta, Georgia

INTRODUCTION

Ovarian carcinoma is the leading cause of gynecological cancer death in the United States [1]. In its early stages, ovarian cancer is difficult to detect and diagnose. This difficulty is underscored by the fact that approximately two-thirds of patients with epithelial carcinoma of the ovary are diagnosed with advanced disease [2]. Even with advanced disease, presurgical assessment and staging is frequently inaccurate [3,4].

The prognosis for patients with ovarian cancer is relatively poor. Most ovarian cancers are rapidly growing and result in large tumor masses that involve other abdominal organs. Residual cancer in the abdominal cavity is not uncommon, even following aggressive surgical resection [5]. To optimize postsurgical adjuvant therapy, accurate assessments of the stage and grade of the tumor, as well as the extent of residual disease, are crucial.

As with initial diagnosis, none of the existing tests [e.g., computed tomographic (CT) scanning] are sufficiently sensitive or specific to rule out the recurrence of tumor [6–8]. However, if CA-125 levels are elevated prior to the original operation, a reelevation of this tumor marker posttherapy is almost always associated with disease. On the other hand, "normal" CA-125 values may be associated with persistent disease in as many as 50% of patients [9]. Second-look surgical exploration is often required to confirm the presence or absence of tumor recurrence.

Thus, there is a need for an accurate, noninvasive diagnostic test for ovarian cancer. An accurate preoperative assessment of the location and extent of tumor spread would be valuable for the initial staging laparotomy. Moreover, such a test would prove useful in monitoring the response to postsurgical adjuvant therapy. It is possible that the need for second-look surgical exploration could be eliminated if the noninvasive test was sufficiently sensitive and specific to detect occult disease.

Monoclonal antibodies directed to tumor-associated antigens and radiolabeled with gamma-emitting radionuclides have been valuable in diagnosing and staging cancer (10–12). B72.3 is a murine monoclonal antibody of the IgG1 subclass that reacts with TAG-72, an antigen reportedly expressed in virtually 100% of ovarian cancer specimens evaluated [13]. This monoclonal antibody exhibits only limited reactivity with most adult normal tissue, including normal ovarian tissue and benign ovarian tumors [14,15], suggesting that it may be an ideal antibody for identifying ovarian carcinomas.

This report describes the results of an open-label multicenter clinical trial in presurgical patients with primary or persistent/recurrent ovarian carcinoma using ^{111}In-CYT-103, an ^{111}In-labeled immunoconjugate of B72.3 prepared using a site-specific conjugation method [16].

MATERIALS AND METHODS
Patient Population

Adult (≥21years) presurgical patients with suspected or biopsy-proven primary or persistent/recurrent epithelial ovarian carcinoma were eligible for participation in this study. Patients who were pregnant, had an expected survival of less than 2 months, had a Karnofsky performance status less than 60%, had a second primary malignancy, had received antitumor therapy during the 4 weeks prior to monoclonal antibody infusion, or had previously received a murine antibody were not eligible for participation. All patients provided written informed consent prior to participation, and the study protocol was approved by the institutional review board at each participating study site.

Study Plan

Baseline evaluations included a medical history, physical examination, standard serum chemistry and hematological laboratory tests and routine urinalysis. Serum measurements of TAG-72 antigen, human antimouse antibody (HAMA) titers (human antibodies to mouse IgG), and CA-125 levels were also performed. TAG-72 determinations were made using the CA-72-4 Radioimmunoassay

(Centocor, Malvern, PA), and HAMA titers were measured using the ImmuSTRIP HAMA Test System (Immunomedics, Warren, NJ). Standard laboratory tests were repeated prior to surgery, and HAMA development was monitored for at least 8 weeks following infusion of ^{111}In-CYT-103.

Within four weeks of surgery, standard imaging tests were performed, including a chest x-ray and CT scan of the abdomen and pelvis. When possible, all CT scans were performed on a high resolution, "third generation" scanner with fast acquisition/reconstruction capabilities, and the minimum acceptable matrix was 320 x 320.

All patients were given a single intravenous infusion of 1 mg of ^{111}In-CYT-103 over approximately 5–10 min. Vital signs were measured at baseline and at specified intervals from 5 to 240 min after initiation of the infusion.

Between 2 and 7 days following ^{111}In-CYT-103 infusion, planar gamma camera images, including anterior and posterior views of the pelvis, abdomen, and thorax, were obtained for each patient using a large-field-of-view gamma camera with a parallel hole medium-energy collimator. Imaging was performed on at least two occasions prior to surgery, not less than 24 hr apart. Single photon emission tomographic (SPECT) imaging of the abdomen and other suspected disease sites was also performed during one of the imaging sessions. Evaluation of the SPECT images indicated they did not contribute to imaging sensitivity beyond that of the planar gamma images, and these results will not be presented.

An on-site nuclear medicine physician interpreted the gamma camera scans prospectively during the study and noted the location of all positively imaged lesions. This information, along with other staging information, including CT scan findings, was discussed with the surgeon preoperatively.

After completion of the two imaging sessions and appraisal of the presurgical findings, surgery was performed. Every attempt was made to confirm the presence of all potential lesions indicated by the preoperative staging modalities with tissue biopsy. Biopsies of tumor tissue were also obtained in the case of unresectable disease. Histopathological examination and immunohistochemical analysis of TAG-72 expression were to be performed on all tumor specimens obtained during surgery or biopsy.

Preparation of ^{111}In-CYT-103

MAb B72.3 was initially prepared by Schlom and co-workers [17] against a membrane-enriched extract of a human metastatic breast carcinoma. Purified, cell culture–produced monoclonal antibody B72.3 was obtained from Celltech (United Kingdom) and site-specifically conjugated with the linker-chelator complex GYK-DTPA to form the immunoconjugate B72.3-GYK-DTPA or CYT-103, as described previously [17]. CYT-103 (Cytogen Corp., Princeton,

NJ) was supplied to each study site in kits containing one vial each of 1 mg of the immunoconjugate at a concentration of 0.5 mg/mL. Radiolabeling with ^{111}In chloride (Amersham Corp.) was performed at each study site. The ^{111}In activity of the administered doses in this study averaged 4.65 mCi (range = 3.27–7.29 mCi).

Efficacy and Safety Analyses

The performance of ^{111}In-CYT-103 immunoscintigraphy was assessed by comparing antibody imaging findings by the on-site readers for each patient with surgical and histopathological findings. In addition, the ability of antibody imaging to correctly identify surgically confirmed tumor lesions was compared with that of CT imaging for each patient having both presurgical assessments ($n = 101$). Finally, the ability of ^{111}In-CYT-103 immunoscintigraphy to correctly identify occult disease was evaluated.

The safety of ^{111}In-CYT-103 infusion was assessed by monitoring adverse events to the infusion and by examining the effects of the immunoconjugate on vital signs and clinical laboratory tests.

RESULTS
Patient Characteristics

A total of 108 patients from 18 study sites satisfied the enrollment criteria and received an infusion of ^{111}In-CYT-103. Five of these patients did not undergo surgery or biopsy. Surgery was postponed in two patients, one patient died prior to surgery, one patient relocated prior to surgery, and surgery was canceled in one patient because of a diagnosis of cryptogenic cirrhosis. Of the 103 patients who underwent surgery or biopsy, 35 were being evaluated for suspicion of primary ovarian adenocarcinoma and 68 were being evaluated for persistent/recurrent disease. The patient population was predominantly white (87%) and the mean age was 57 years.

A postsurgical diagnosis of ovarian adenocarcinoma was made for 71 patients and benign ovarian tumors for 10 patients. One patient had a borderline ovarian malignancy and two others had nonadenocarcinoma malignancies. The remaining 19 patients were tumor-free at surgery.

^{111}In-CYT-103 Imaging Sensitivity and Specificity

Table 1 summarizes the sensitivity and specificity of ^{111}In-CYT-103 immunoscintigraphy as assessed by the on-site reader. Antibody imaging correctly identified at least one surgically confirmed tumor in 68% of patients with ovarian

Table 1 Sensitivity and Specificity of ^{111}In-CYT-103
Immunoscintigraphy for Ovarian Adenocarcinoma

% (number) of patients correctly diagnosed by ^{111}In-CYT-103 imaging	
Patient population	Per-patient analysis
Confirmed adenocarcinoma	68% (47/71)
Benign ovarian tumor	50% (5/10)
Tumor-free	58% (11/19)
All patients	64% (64/100)
Lesion type	Per-lesion analysis
Confirmed adenocarcinoma	59% (62/105)
Unconfirmed lesion[a]	19

[a]False positive radiolocalizations on antibody scans at sites found
to be free of tumor at surgery.

adenocarcinoma. Following completion of the study, the planar gamma images
were also read by two blinded nuclear medicine experts.

As shown in Table 1, a total of 19 areas of abnormal radiolocalization
were considered to be compatible with tumor by the on-site readers and were
subsequently determined to be nonadenocarcinoma tissue upon histopathological
analysis. Of these 19 false positive radiolocalizations, three of the tissues were
histopathologically normal, five were benign ovarian tumors, one was a nonadenocarcinoma malignancy, and the remaining 10 contained other types
of abnormal, nonmalignant tissues (e.g., inflammatory tissue). Ten of the
nineteen tissues were examined for TAG-72 expression, and none were found
to contain TAG-72, the antigen target of ^{111}In-CYT-103.

A number of variables were evaluated with respect to the sensitivity of
^{111}In-CYT-103 imaging of ovarian adenocarcinoma. These evaluations are
summarized in Table 2. The sensitivity of antibody imaging tended to be higher
for patients with primary disease than for those with persistent/recurrent disease;
the difference in imaging sensitivity for primary versus persistent/recurrent
disease was statistically significant ($p = 0.008$). In an attempt to explain the
relatively higher sensitivity of antibody imaging for primary ovarian
adenocarcinoma, the influence of tumor size on imaging sensitivity was explored.
As shown in Table 2, there was a statistically significant increase in antibody
imaging sensitivity as tumor size increased ($p = 0.001$). Comparing tumor
size among patients with primary or persistent/recurrent disease revealed a
preponderance of smaller lesions (≥ 2 cm) among patients with persistent/

Table 2 Variables Affecting Sensitivity of ^{111}In-CYT-103 Immunoscintigraphy in Detecting Ovarian Adenocarcinomas

% (number of patients or lesions correctly diagnosed/detected by ^{111}In-CYT-103 imaging	
Disease state[a]	
Primary	95% (18/19)*
Recurrent	58% (30/52)
Tumor size[b,c]	
Microscopic	8% (1/13)
Miliary (<0.5 cm)	59% (10/17)
≥0.5 cm to ≤2 cm	47% (8/17)
>2 cm	81% (17/21)*
Serum TAG-72 titer[a]	
Not recorded	78% (7/9)
Negative (<10 U/ml)	64% (30/47)
Positive (≥10 U/ml)	73% (11/15)
Prior chemotherapy[a]	
Yes	59% (30/51)
No	90% (18/20)*
TAG-72 antigen expression of tumor[c]	
Not done	39% (11/28)
0 – <5%	31% (4/13)
5 – <40%	73% (35/48)
40 – 80%	75% (12/16)

[a]Per-patient analysis.
[b]Tumor size recorded for only 68 of 105 adenocarcinoma lesions.
[c]Per-lesion analysis.
*Statistically significant ($p \leq 0.05$) difference in sensitivity between variable categories.

recurrent ovarian adenocarcinoma (75%). In contrast, only 42% of patients with primary ovarian adenocarcinoma in this study had lesions ≤ 2 cm. When only patients with lesions > 2 cm were considered, the imaging sensitivity was 79% for patients with persistent/recurrent disease and 86% for patients with primary disease.

Although there was a statistically significant association between prior chemotherapy and increased antibody imaging sensitivity ($p = 0.03$), this effect cannot be separated from the difference in imaging sensitivity between patients with primary and persistent/recurrent disease. All but one patient with persistent/recurrent ovarian carcinoma had previous chemotherapy.

Serum TAG-72 titers were measured prior to infusion of ^{111}In-CYT-103 for 62 of the 71 patients with surgically confirmed ovarian adenocarcinoma; 15 of these patients had positive serum titers (≥ 10 U/liter). Although the presence of the TAG-72 antigen in serum might have been expected to reduce tumor localization of the antibody, there was no significant difference in antibody imaging sensitivity in patients with positive or negative serum titers of TAG-72.

Of the 77 surgically confirmed tumor lesions that were evaluated for expression of TAG-72, 64 were found to contain the antigen on the sections examined. As expected, the sensitivity of ^{111}In-CYT-103 imaging increased with increasing antigen content (see Table 2). This increase was statistically significant ($p = 0.02$).

^{111}In-CYT-103 Immunoscintigraphy Versus CT

All but 2 of the 103 patients who underwent surgery or biopsy following ^{111}In-CYT-103 infusion had CT scans performed as part of their presurgical workup. The performance of CT imaging and ^{111}In-CYT-103 imaging in the 101 patients who were evaluated by both imaging modalities is presented in Table 3. A comparison of the two imaging modalities reveals that the sensitivity of ^{111}In-CYT-103 imaging (48/70; 69%) for detecting ovarian adenocarcinoma was greater than that of CT imaging (31/70; 44%); however, the per-patient specificity of CT imaging (22/28; 79%) was higher than that of antibody imaging (15/28; 54%).

A further comparison of the two imaging modalities considered their performance in individual patients. Of the 70 patients with surgically confirmed ovarian adenocarcinoma who were evaluated by both CT and ^{111}In-CYT-103 imaging, tumor lesions were correctly identified by both modalities in 29 patients. ^{111}In-CYT-103 imaging correctly detected tumor lesions in an additional 19 patients who had negative CT scans; however, CT scans detected tumor lesions in only two patients with negative antibody images.

Carcinomatosis was present in 39 of the 71 patients with surgically confirmed ovarian carcinoma; 38 of these patients were evaluated by both CT and antibody

Table 3 Sensitivity and Specificity of ^{111}In-CYT-103 Immunoscintigraphy and Computed Tomography (CT) Imaging for Ovarian Adenocarcinomas

Imaging performance parameter	Disease status	% (no.) patients/lesions correctly diagnosed	
		Antibody imaging	CT imaging
Sensitivity			
Per-patient	Primary	95% (18/19)	84% (16/19)
Analysis	Recurrent	59% (30/51)	29% (15/51)
Per-lesion	Primary	81% (21/26)	77% (20/26)
Analysis	Recurrent	53% (41/78)	23% (18/78)
Specificity Per-patient:			
Benign ovarian	Primary	50% (5/10)	60% (6/10)
Tumors	Recurrent	–	–
Tumor-free	Primary	50% (2/4)	50% (2/4)
	Recurrent	57% (8/14)	100% (14/14)
No. false positive lesions	All patients	15	14

imaging. The overall detection rate for carcinomatosis by ^{111}In-CYT-103 imaging was 71% (27 of 38 patients), and for CT imaging it was 45% (17 OF 38 patients). Planar gamma camera images for a patient whose antibody images confirmed the presence of carcinomatosis, but whose CT scan was negative, are shown in Figure 1.

These results indicate that ^{111}In-CYT-103 immunoscintigraphy is more sensitive than CT imaging in presurgical patients with ovarian adenocarcinoma.

Detection of Occult Disease by ^{111}In-CYT-103 Immunoscintigraphy

^{111}In-CYT-103 immunoscintigraphy detected occult disease in 20 of the 71 patients (28%) with surgically confirmed ovarian adenocarcinoma. Seventeen of these patients were being evaluated prior to restaging laparotomy. A total of 24 lesions were detected by antibody imaging in the 20 patients with occult disease (Table 4); 12 (50%) of these lesions were < 2 cm in size. Six of the twenty

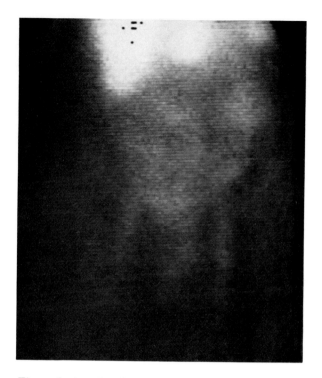

Figure 1 Anterior planar gamma camera images of a patient scheduled for secon-look laparotomy. The patient's presurgical workup, including a CT scan, was negative for malignant disease. The antibody images were consistent with carcinomatosis. At surgery, the patient was found to have extensive disease recurrence, including tumor seeding of the mesentery, abdominal wall, and pelvis.

Table 4 Location of Occult Disease Lesions Detected by [111] In-CYT-103 Immunoscintigraphy

Location	No. of occult lesions
Abdomen	3
Carcinomatosis	8
Colon, ascending	1
Cul-de-sac	1
Large or small bowel mesentery	5
Omentum	4
Periaortic lymph node	1
Small bowel	1

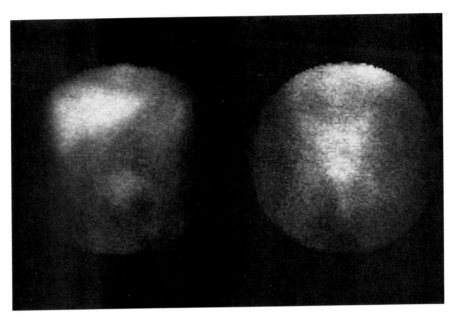

Figure 2 Anterior planar gamma camera images of a patient evaluated for residual/recurrent disease. In addition to localizing the patient's known pelvic recurrence, the antibody images detected occult tumor deposits on the anterior abdominal wall and in the mesentery. The antibody scan findings were confirmed at surgery.

patients with antibody-detected occult disease had an otherwise negative presurgical workup and a normal serum CA-125 level, suggesting that ^{111}In CYT-103 immunoscintigraphy may be particularly useful for the earlier detection of disease or disease recurrence in this population of ovarian cancer patients. An example of a patient whose antibody images detected the presence of occult disease (single malignant tumor nodule in the small bowel) that was otherwise undetected on presurgical workup is illustrated in Figure 2. Of particular note, ^{111}In-CYT-103 detected carcinomatosis in 8 of the 20 patients with occult disease; other diagnostic tests, including CT scans, have shown poor sensitivity for diffuse miliary disease.

Safety of ^{111}In-CYT-103 Infusion

Adverse Events

Three of the 108 patients (2.8%) who received ^{111}In-CYT-103 infusion experienced adverse events that were considered by the investigator to be at least possibly related to the study medication. Subsequent analysis of these adverse events revealed that infusion of ^{111}In-CYT-103 was probably related to only one of these events. One patient experienced a mild elevation in blood pressure (162/120 mm Hg) 1 hr postinfusion; prior to infusion, her blood pressure was 134/88 mm Hg. Her blood pressure was still elevated 2 hr postinfusion.

A second patient experienced a reduction in blood pressure considered possibly related to ^{111}In-CYT-103 infusion; however, this patient had a high preinfusion blood pressure (180/90 mm Hg), and the reductions observed postinfusion (125/75–130/80 mm Hg) were thought to reflect normalization following preinfusion anxiety. Severe shaking chills, knee joint pain, back pain, ankle tenderness, erythema, and fever were observed in a third patient 5 days following ^{111}In-CYT-103 infusion. Although these events were initially thought to be possibly related to study medication, the patient was subsequently found to have staphyloccal septicemia related to an infected catheter.

No clinically significant trends were noted for changes in vital signs or clinical laboratory tests following ^{111}In-CYT-103 infusion.

HAMA Titers

HAMA titers were evaluated preinfusion and for up to 8 weeks postinfusion for each patient. The frequency of HAMA development following ^{111}In-CYT-103 infusion was calculated by determining the ratio of HAMA-positive patients to that of HAMA-positive and HAMA-negative (HAMA titer < 0.4 μg/ml for $\geq$ 4 weeks postinfusion) patients. As of this report, 44 of the 65 patients evaluated for $\geq$ 4 weeks postinfusion were HAMA negative; thus, the frequency of HAMA development following ^{111}In-CYT-103 infusion in this study was 32% (21/65). For most of these patients (90.5%), the positive titers were first observed between 1 and 4 weeks postinfusion, and the mean peak HAMA titer measurement was 2.03 μg/ml.

DISCUSSION

The results of this multicenter trial suggest that ^{111}In-CYT-103 immunoscintigraphy may be a valuable whole-body, presurgical diagnostic imaging test for patients with suspected primary or persistent/recurrent ovarian adenocarcinoma. The sensitivity of ^{111}In-CYT-103 immunoscintigraphy for correctly identifying patients with ovarian adenocarcinoma was 68%. ^{111}In-CYT-103 immunoscintigraphy was more sensitive than CT imaging in presurgical patients with ovarian adenocarcinoma, as indicated not only by a greater overall sensitivity for detecting tumor lesions but by correctly identifying tumor lesions in multiple patients with negative CT scans. Furthermore, ^{111}In-CYT-103 immunoscintigraphy was successful in identifying occult disease in 20 patients (28%) with surgically confirmed ovarian adenocarcinoma. Among these 20 patients with occult disease correctly identified by antibody imaging were six patients with an otherwise negative presurgical workup and a normal serum CA-125 level. These results suggest that ^{111}In-CYT-103 immunoscintigraphy may be particularly useful in the earlier detection of disease or disease recurrence in patients with ovarian cancer.

The sensitivity of ^{111}In-CYT-103 immunoscintigraphy was influenced both by the size of the tumor lesion and by the tumor TAG-72 antigen expression. The sensitivity of antibody imaging was 47–59% for tumor lesions $\leq$ 2 cm but was over 80% for lesions > 2 cm. Additionally, the sensitivity of ^{111}In-CYT-103 immunoscintigraphy was higher for tumor lesions demonstrating greater TAG-72 antigen expression. Of particular note, serum titers of TAG-72 had no influence on the sensitivity of antibody imaging in this study.

The overall sensitivity of ^{111}In-CYT-103 immunoscintigraphy in ovarian adenocarcinoma compares favorably to reports of its use in colorectal cancer. The sensitivity of ^{111}In-CYT-103 immunoscintigraphy in colorectal cancer has been reported to be approximately 70% [18,19].

The sensitivity of ^{111}In-CYT-103 immunoscintigraphy in ovarian adenocarcinoma also compares favorably to reports of immunoscintigraphy performed using other monoclonal antibodies [20]. A common finding in such studies is a less than optimal specificity. A similar finding was evident in this study using ^{111}In-CYT-103 immunoscintigraphy. These data suggest that, in the absence of other presurgical diagnostic information, antibody imaging can only suggest the differential diagnosis of benign versus malignant disease in patients with an undiagnosed pelvic mass. Furthermore, a negative monoclonal antibody scan should not be used to defer second-look surgical exploration when it is otherwise indicated. In this regard, ^{111}In-CYT-103 immunoscintigraphy shares certain of the performance characteristics of other, nonsurgical diagnostic and staging modalities for ovarian carcinoma [3].

In summary, the ability of ^{111}In-CYT-103 immunoscintigraphy to correctly detect primary and recurrent ovarian tumors – including occult lesions – combined with its favorable safety profile, indicate that it should be a useful addition to the presurgical evaluation of patients with ovarian adenocarcinoma.

ACKNOWLEDGMENTS

Appreciation is expressed to the following clinical investigators, who, in addition to the author, participated in the ^{111}In-CYT-103 multicenter clinical trial: Earl Surwit, M.D. (University of Arizona); J. Gale Katterhagen, M.D. (Memorial Cancer Center, Springfield, IL); Jon A. Kotler, M.D. (Cleveland Clinic, Florida); Edith P. Mitchell, M.D. (University of Missouri); Ruth Oratz, M.D. (New York University Medical Center); Larry L. Copeland, M.D. (Ohio State University);

William J. Mann, M.D. (State University of New York at Stony Brook); Holly H. Gallion, M.D. (University of Kentucky); David N. Krag, M.D. (University of California at Davis); Gary Purnell, M.D. (University of Arkansas for Medical Sciences); Gregorio Delgado, M.D. (Georgetown University Hospital); Aldo N. Serafini, M.D. (University of Miami School of Medicine); Edgardo L. Yordan, Jr., M.D. (Rush–Presbyterian–St. Luke's Medical Center, Illinois); Bruce R. Line, M.D. and John H. Malfetano, M.D. (Albany Medical College, New York); George Q. Mills, M.D. (Our Lady of the Lake Regional Medical Center, Louisiana); Howard D. Homesley, M.D. (Bowman Gray School of Medicine, North Carolina); and W. Newlon Tauxe, M.D., and Geoffrey Levine, Ph.D. (Presbyterian–University Hospital, Pittsburgh, PA). This multicenter study was supported by a grant from CYTOGEN Corporation (Princeton, NJ).

REFERENCES

1. Silverberg E, Boung C, Squires TS. Cancer statistics, 1990. CA 1990; 40:9–26.
2. Katz ME, Schwartz PE, Kopp DS, et al. Epithelial carcinoma of the ovaries: current strategies. Ann Intern Med 1981; 195:98–111.
3. McGowan L, Parent Lesher L, Norris HL, Barnett M. Misstaging of ovarian cancer. Obstet Gynecol 1985; 65:568–72.
4. Piver MS. Ovarian carcinoma: a decade of progress. Cancer 1984; 54:2706–15.
5. Redman JR, Petroni RZ, Sargo PE. Prognostic factors in advanced ovarian carcinoma. J Clin Oncol 1986; 4:513–23.
6. Young RC, Fuks Z, Hoskins WJ. Cancer of the ovary. In: Cancer: Principles and Practices of Oncology. Philadelphia:Lippincott, 1989:1162–96.
7. Shepherd JH, Granowska M, Britton FE, et al. Tumour-associated monoclonal antibodies for the diagnosis and assessment of ovarian cancer. Br J Obstet Gynaecol 1987; 94:160–7.
8. Silverman PM, Osbourne M, Dunnick NR, Bandy LC. CT prior to second-look operation in ovarian cancer. Am J Roentgenol 1988; 150:829–32.
9. Ruben SC, Hoskins WJ, Haken TB, et al. Serum CA 125 levels and surgical findings in patients undergoing secondary operations for epithelial ovarian cancer. Am J Obstet Gynecol 1989; 160:667–71.
10. Haller DG. Monoclonal antibody imaging in the management of patients with colorectal cancer. J Clin Oncol 1988; 6:1213–15.
11. Larson SM. Lymphoma, melanoma, colon cancer: diagnosis and treatment with radiolabeled monoclonal antibodies. Radiology 1987; 165:297–304.
12. Byers VS, Baldwin RW. Therapeutic strategies with monoclonal antibodies and immunoconjugates. Immunology 1988; 65:329–35.
13. Thor A, Ohuchi N, Szpak CA, Johnston WW, Schlom J. Distribution of onco-fetal antigen tumor-associated glycoprotein-72 defined by monoclonal antibody B72.3. Cancer Res 1986; 46:3118–24.

14. Thor A, Gorstein F, Ohuchi N, et al. Tumor-associated glycoprotein (TAG-72) in ovarian carcinomas defined by monoclonal antibody B72.3. J Natl Cancer Inst 1986; 76:995-1006.
15. Thor A, Viglione MJ, Murar R, et al. Monoclonal antibody B72.3 reactivity with human endometrium: a study of normal and malignant tissues. Int J Gynecol Pathol 1987; 6:235-47.
16. Rodwell JD, Alvarez VL, Lee C, et al. Site-specific covalent modification of monoclonal antibodies: in vitro and in vivo evaluations. Proc Natl Acad Sci USA 1986; 83:2632-6.
17. Colcher D, Horan Hand P, Nuti M, et al. A spectrum of monoclonal antibodies reactive with mammary tumor cells. Proc Natl Acad Sci USA 1981; 78:3199-3202.
18. Maguire RT, Schmelter RF, Pascucci VL, Conklin JJ. Immunoscintigraphy of colorectal adenocarcinoma: results with site-specifically radiolabeled B72.3 (^{111}In-CYT-103). Antibody Immunoconjugates Radiopharmaceut 1989; 2:257-69.
19. Doerr RJ, Abdel-Nabi H, Krag D, Mitchell E. Radiolabeled antibody imaging in the management of colorectal cancer: results of a multicenter clinical study. Ann Surg 1990 (submitted).
20. Thor AD, Edgerton SM. Monoclonal antibodies reactive with human breast or ovarian carcinoma: in vivo applications. Semin Nucl Med 1989; 19:295-308.

8

Impact of ^{111}In-CYT-103 on the Surgical Management of Patients with Ovarian Cancer

Earl A. Surwit

University of Arizona, Tucson, Arizona

INTRODUCTION

Although ovarian cancer ranks second in incidence among cancers of the female reproductive tract, with approximately 20,000 new cases diagnosed each year in the United States, it causes more deaths than all other gynecological malignancies combined [1]. Overall, the 5-year survival rate of ovarian cancer patients is 38%. A number of factors contribute to this low survival rate, including stage of disease at presentation, accuracy of intraoperative staging, and completeness of the initial surgical procedure [2–5]. Because of the insidious nature of early ovarian carcinoma, the initial diagnosis is often delayed, with over 60% of patients presenting with regional metastases and/or extrapelvic disease [4].

Diagnosis and Staging of Ovarian Cancer

After the initial discovery of a pelvic mass, which is generally made by pelvic examination, numerous presurgical procedures, including intravenous pyelogram, barium enema, cystoscopy, proctosigmoidoscopy, ultrasound, computed tomography (CT), and abdominal and chest x-rays, may be employed in an attempt to obtain a differential diagnosis. However, the major value of most of these tests is in ruling out nonmalignant pelvic disorders, and none is reliable for the definitive assignment of a benign or malignant etiology for an undiagnosed pelvic mass or for the accurate and complete staging of ovarian neoplasms [5,6].

Because of the limitations of existing diagnostic modalities, the initial diagnosis and staging of ovarian carcinoma generally requires surgical and histopathological data. Unfortunately, the results of retrospective evaluations of intraoperative staging procedures indicate that the majority of patients have surgical evaluations that are inadequate for accurate staging [7,8]. In one series of 291 patients, only 80 (28%) were considered to have the correct stage of disease recorded after their initial exploratory surgery [9]. In this series, the accuracy of the staging laparotomy was dependent upon the expertise of the operating surgeon, with gynecological oncologists performing adequate surgical evaluations in 97% of the patients, as compared with 52% and 35% rates for obstetricians/gynecologists and general surgeons, respectively.

The utility of available diagnostic modalities is also limited in the management of ovarian cancer patients following their initial surgical procedure. The potential role for these tests in this setting includes monitoring the response to chemotherapy or radiation therapy. Various diagnostic studies, including liver function tests, barium enema, intravenous pyelography, CT imaging, and measurement of serum levels of the tumor marker CA-125, are used for monitoring the response to adjuvant therapy. Although each of these tests may be of value in confirming a recurrence, none is sensitive and specific enough to rule out tumor recurrence. The documented complete remission rate in patients undergoing second-look surgery is approximately half the complete clinical response rate predicted prior to surgery [9]. Therefore, as with the initial diagnostic workup for ovarian cancer, surgical evaluation is frequently required for monitoring antitumor therapy, for posttreatment restaging and debulking, and to assist in the selection of second-line therapy.

Requirements for New Nonsurgical Diagnostic Approaches for Ovarian Cancer

The need for improved nonsurgical diagnostic and staging modalities for ovarian cancer is apparent in view of the limitations of the existing diagnostic tests. New techniques would be valuable both for the evaluation of an unknown pelvic mass (i.e., primary disease) and for the assessment of residual or recurrent disease after completion of first-line therapy. To significantly contribute to management decisions for patients with primary or recurrent ovarian cancer, however, different performance characteristics are required of a diagnostic and staging test.

A key component in the decision-making process for presurgical patients with an undiagnosed pelvic mass is the ability to distinguish between benign and malignant disease. A diagnostic modality with adequate specificity could assist in the management of such patients because accurate information concerning the malignant etiology of a pelvic mass would permit appropriate referral to a surgical oncologist for the performance of the initial staging laparotomy. The importance of an accurate and complete initial surgical evaluation has been discussed above. The sensitivity of the diagnostic test for ovarian tumor lesions is also important for the evaluation of patients with primary disease. The identification of metastatic tumor deposits, especially the miliary and microscopic disease that characterizes advanced ovarian carcinoma, could help optimize the initial surgical procedure. By directing the removal of otherwise occult disease, especially lesions located outside the proposed surgical field, such a diagnostic test could lead to more thorough debulking and, therefore, improve the response to postsurgical treatment and potentially improve survival.

In patients with known ovarian carcinoma who are being evaluated for potential recurrence after completion of adjuvant therapy, accurate assessment of the presence and extent of disease is critical to subsequent management decisions. The detection of tumor recurrence in this patient population might allow the use of laparoscopy or fine-needle biopsy to confirm the diagnosis, thereby avoiding the morbidity and expense associated with second-look surgery, the value of which remains controversial (9,10). Since ovarian cancer primarily affects elderly individuals, morbid and/or toxic medical or surgical therapies should be avoided unless they are absolutely necessary. A sensitive diagnostic test used in conjunction with the limited surgical procedures noted above could help to make decisions concerning the discontinuation of toxic chemotherapeutic regimens and/or the institution of second-line treatments, including intraperitoneal chemotherapy.

¹¹¹In-CYT-103 Immunoscintigraphy in the Management of Ovarian Cancer

Monoclonal antibodies directed to tumor-associated antigens and labeled with gamma-emitting radionuclides have been utilized for the diagnosis and staging of malignant tumors [11–13]. Several radiolabeled monoclonal antibodies are being investigated for the detection of ovarian carcinoma [14–19]. The preliminary findings of these investigations have demonstrated that monoclonal antibody imaging has the potential to detect occult tumor lesions, including carcinomatosis, in patients with ovarian cancer. These encouraging results suggest that immunoscintigraphy using radiolabeled monoclonal antibodies may be useful both for the initial diagnosis and staging of this disease and for the evaluation of residual disease after adjuvant treatment and prior to second-look laparotomy.

We previously conducted a preliminary investigation of ^{111}In-CYT-103, an ^{111}In-labeled immunoconjugate of monoclonal antibody B72.3 [20]. The potential utility of the B72.3 antibody has been suggested by its reactivity with ovarian neoplasms and its successful use as an immunoscintigraphic agent for ovarian and other reactive adenocarcinomas [19,21]. ^{111}In-CYT-103 differs from other radiolabeled conjugates of B72.3 in that the attachment of the radionuclide occurs exclusively on the oligosaccharide moiety of the antibody molecule [22]. This approach offers an advantage over random attachment methods because modification of the antibody occurs at a site distal to the antigen-combining site. Radiolabeled immunoconjugates prepared by the site-specific method have a high specific activity and retain the immunoreactivity of the unmodified antibody [22].

In our initial ^{111}In-CYT-103 clinical trial, 19 women with primary or recurrent ovarian carcinoma were administered single intravenous (i.v.) doses of the radiolabeled immunoconjugate [20]. Gamma camera imaging was performed within 7 days after ^{111}In-CYT-103 administration and prior to laparotomy. The results of immunoscintigraphy were compared with the surgical and histopathological findings to determine imaging efficacy. The results of this preliminary investigation indicated that ^{111}In-CYT-103 could be safely administered to patients with ovarian carcinoma, and that immunoscintigraphy with this agent detected tumor in 77% of the patients (10 of 13) with surgically confirmed disease. The detection of occult lesions, i.e., tumor deposits that were not detected by other presurgical diagnostic tests, in five patients suggested that this radiolabeled immunoconjugate has the ability to provide information useful in the clinical management of ovarian cancer patients. Moreover, the antibody scan findings were reported to increase the surgeon's knowledge of the patients' disease for 6 of the 19 patients (32%) evaluated [20].

As a result of these encouraging preliminary findings, a multicenter ^{111}In-CYT-103 clinical trial was conducted in patients with known or suspected primary or recurrent ovarian carcinoma [23]. This study provided a definitive demonstration of the imaging efficacy of the radiolabeled immunoconjugate and, importantly, helped to define the utility of this agent in the management of various subsets of ovarian carcinoma patients. The safety and imaging efficacy results of the multicenter trial have been presented elsewhere in this book [23]. In this chapter, we present an evaluation of the potential effect of immunoscintigraphy with ^{111}In-CYT-103 on the management of ovarian cancer patients.

METHODS

The potential impact of antibody imaging with ^{111}In-CYT-103 was assessed during a multicenter clinical trial conducted at 18 study sites. At each center, the study protocol was approved by the appropriate institutional review board, and each patient enrolled in the trial provided written informed consent. The design and the safety and imaging efficacy results of this multicenter study have been described previously [23]. Briefly, presurgical patients with known or suspected primary or recurrent ovarian carcinoma were administered single intravenous infusions of 1 mg of CYT-103, monoclonal antibody B72.3 site-specifically conjugated to the linker-chelator, glycyl-tyrosyl-(N,ϵ-diethylenetri-aminepentaacetic acid)-lysine, radiolabeled with approximately 5 mCi of ^{111}In. Gamma camera imaging, including both planar and single photon emission computed tomographic (SPECT) studies, was performed between 2 and 7 days after administration of ^{111}In-CYT-103. Other required presurgical diagnostic tests included a chest x-ray and a CT scan with contrast of the abdomen and pelvis. The imaging efficacy of ^{111}In-CYT-103 immunoscintigraphy was determined by a comparison of the antibody scan results with the surgical and histopathological findings.

The potential impact of ^{111}In-CYT-103 immunoscintigraphy on the surgical management of the patients was assessed through a series of questions completed by the clinical investigators at various points during each patient's participation in the trial. One set of questions was to be answered after the antibody scan findings had been reviewed but prior to surgery. At this time, the investigator was asked to respond to the following questions.

1. Did the monoclonal antibody scan change your estimate of the extent of disease?
2. Would the results of the monoclonal antibody scan potentially change the surgical plan?
3. Based on the findings of the monoclonal antibody scan, were further preoperative studies suggested?

For each affirmative response to the above questions, the investigators were asked to provide an explanation.

A final assessment of the potential effect of the antibody scan findings on the patient's management was made after the surgical and histopathological results were known. For this assessment, the investigators were required to rate the impact of antibody imaging as either very beneficial, beneficial, no effect, negative, or very negative for each patient. The investigators were given no guidance or predetermined criteria for the assignment of the rating scores. Comments explaining the ratings they selected for each patient were requested. The investigators' assessments before and after the surgical and histopathological results were compared to determine their correlation.

In addition to the investigators' assessment of the potential impact of antibody imaging on the management of individual patients, the antibody imaging performance data from the clinical trial were examined to identify subsets of patients for whom this diagnostic test appeared to be particularly valuable.

For this evaluation, an attempt was made to determine the relationship between the antibody imaging performance results and patient management assessment. Utilizing the immunoscintigraphic findings, as well as a comparison of the results of antibody imaging with the results of other presurgical diagnostic tests, the potential impact of the new technology on the management of the various subgroups of patients was examined.

RESULTS
Patient Population, Surgical Findings, and Antibody Imaging Results

Data are presented for the patients enrolled in the multicenter trial who received ^{111}In-CYT-103 infusions, completed gamma camera imaging studies, and, subsequently, underwent surgical exploration. As shown in Table 1, this population included 103 patients. Thirty-five patients were evaluated for primary ovarian carcinoma (i.e., undiagnosed pelvic mass) and 68 were evaluated for the potential recurrence of ovarian carcinoma. The population was predominantly white and had a mean age of 57 years. The patients with suspected primary disease were significantly ($p < 0.05$; t test) older than those evaluated for residual or recurrent disease.

Table 2 summarizes the performance results for ^{111}In-CYT-103 immunoscintigraphy in this patient population. As shown, antibody imaging sensitivity was especially high in patients with primary ovarian carcinoma. The sensitivity differences between the patients with primary versus recurrent ovarian carcinoma

Table 1 Demographic Characteristics of the Patients

Parameter	Primary disease	Recurrent disease	All patients
No. of patients	35	68	103
Age (years)			
Mean	60	55	57
Range	34–84	26–78	26–84
Race			
White	30 (86%)	60 (88%)	90 (87%)
Black	4 (11%)	2 (3%)	6 (6%)
Hispanic	0	3 (4%)	3 (3%)
Other	1 (3%)	3 (4%)	4 (4%)

Table 2 Summary of Performance of ^{111}In-CYT-103 Immunoscintigraphy

Antibody imaging performance parameters	No. (%) of patients by presurgical diagnosis		
	Primary disease[a]	Recurrent disease	All patients
Sensitivity in patients with surgically confirmed ovarian carcinoma	18/19 (95%)	30/52 (58%)	48/71 (68%)
Specificity in patients who did not have ovarian carcinoma at surgery	7/15 (47%)	10/16 (63%)	17/31 (55%)
Positive predictive value	18/26 (69%)	30/36 (83%)	–
Negative predictive value	7/8 (88%)	10/32 (31%)	–

[a]Excludes data for one patient with a presurgical diagnosis of primary ovarian cancer. Surgical pathological findings revealed a borderline malignancy (serous papillary tumor with borderline features), which was detected by antibody imaging.

were statistically significant ($p \leq 0.05$; chi square). This resulted, in large part, from the difference in the sizes of the tumor lesions observed in the two groups of patients, specifically the preponderance of smaller (≤ 2 cm) lesions in patients with recurrent or residual ovarian cancer.

An important aspect of the imaging performance findings was the ability of immunoscintigraphy to detect adenocarcinoma lesions that had been missed by other presurgical diagnostic and staging modalities. Antibody imaging detected such occult disease in 20 of the 71 patients (28%) with surgically confirmed ovarian carcinoma. In these 20 patients, 17 of whom were being evaluated prior to restaging laparotomy, antibody imaging detected 24 tumor lesions that were not detected by physical examination or by other diagnostic tests conducted prior to ^{111}In-CYT-103 immunoscintigraphy (see Chapter 7). Twelve of the 20 patients had no evidence of disease on pelvic examination or by other presurgical diagnostic imaging tests. Importantly, 5 of the 17 patients evaluated for recurrence had an otherwise negative presurgical workup and a normal serum CA-125 level. Thus, in this subset of patients, immunoscintigraphy provided the only presurgical indication of residual ovarian adenocarcinoma. These results suggest that antibody imaging with ^{111}In–CYT–103 may be particularly useful for the earlier detection of disease recurrence in this population of ovarian cancer patients.

Identification of previously occult tumor lesions by antibody imaging clearly enhanced the surgeon's knowledge of the presence and extent of disease in this subset of patients. However, the actual impact of the discovery of occult lesions on the subsequent management of the patient varies with the location of the lesion, the status of the patient's disease, and the influence of such a positive finding on the patient's treatment plan. The implications of the localization of occult disease by ^{111}In-CYT-103 immunoscintigraphy on the surgical management of these patients will be discussed below.

Antibody Imaging: Potential Impact on Patient Management

As discussed, pre and postsurgical assessments of the impact of ^{111}In-CYT-103 immunoscintigraphy on patient management were made by the clinical investigators. Presurgical evaluations were completed for 102 of the 103 patients, and postsurgical data were available for the entire study population. A summary of the investigators' responses to specific questions, which comprised these assessments, is shown in Table 3. In their utilization of the antibody imaging results prior to surgery, the investigators indicated that these findings changed their estimate of the extent of disease for 27% of the patients and potentially changed the proposed surgical plan for 16%; the antibody scan results did not suggest additional noninvasive preoperative diagnostic tests for any of the patients.

After the surgical and histopathological findings were known, the investigators were asked to rate the overall contribution of the antibody scan results to the management of each patient. These ratings provided a final assessment of the overall positive or negative impact of ^{111}In-CYT-103 for each patient. As shown in Table 3, the antibody scan findings were considered beneficial or very beneficial for 27% of the patients and negative or very negative for 2%, whereas for the remainder of the patients (71%), the results of antibody imaging were considered to have had neither a beneficial nor a negative effect. Sixteen of sixty-eight patients (24%) with recurrent disease and 12 of 35 (34%) with primary disease were assigned ratings of beneficial or very beneficial, whereas both patients assigned ratings of negative or very negative were patients with an undiagnosed pelvic mass who were evaluated for suspicion of ovarian carcinoma.

Antibody Imaging Performance Versus Patient Management Impact

Beneficial and very beneficial ratings were generally assigned in cases where the antibody scans provided accurate diagnostic information, whereas the two negative or very negative ratings were associated with false positive antibody

Table 3 Investigators' Responses Regarding the Patient Management Impact of Antibody (MAb) Imaging

Presurgical Assessment

	Responses: no. (%) of patients		
Question	Yes	No	Not Recorded
1. Did the MAb scan findings change estimate of extent of disease?	28/103 (27%)	74/103	1/103
2. Would the MAb scan findings potentially change the proposed surgical plan?	16/103 (16%)	86/103	1/103
3. Did the MAb scan findings suggest additional preoperative diagnostic studies?	0/103 (0%)	102/103	1/103

Postsurgical Assessment

Effect of the MAb scan findings on management of the patient	No. (%) of patients	
Very beneficial	6/103	(6%)
Beneficial	22/103	(21%)
No effect	73/103	(71%)
Negative	1/103	(1%)
Very negative	1/103	(1%)

Comparison Between Postsurgical and Presurgical Responses

		No. with positive responses to presurgical questions			
Postsurgical response	Total No.	MAb changed either extent of disease or surgical plan		MAb changed both extent of disease and surgical plan	
Very beneficial	6	5/6	(83%)	1/6	(17%)
Beneficial	22	13/22	(59%)	5/22	(23%)
No effect	71	16/71	(23%)	2/71	(3%)
Negative	1	0/1	(0%)	0/1	(0%)
Very negative	1	1/1	(100%)	1/1	(100%)

Table 4 Antibody (MAb) Imaging Performance in Patients Assigned Beneficial or Very Beneficial Patient Management Ratings

MAb scan findings	No. of patients
1. Detected occult disease and provided only positive presurgical finding in patients with surgically confirmed carcinoma	
Microscopic disease in abdomen	1
Tumor nodule in small bowel	1
Miliary disease in mesentery of small and large bowel	1
2. Detected occult carcinoma lesions, which were confirmed at surgery	
Carcinomatosis	2
Lymph node metastasis	1
Miliary implants in omentum	2
Metastases in colon and omentum	1
3. Confirmed positive findings of other diagnostic tests; findings were subsequently confirmed at surgery	
Lymph node metastasis	2
Pelvic tumor	3
Carcinomatosis	7
4. Negative findings in patients who were tumor free at surgery	2
5. Negative findings or scan consistent with benign cyst in patients found to have benign ovarian tumors	2
6. Other equivocal findings that resulted in beneficial ratings	2
Indeterminate radiolocalization in area of surgically confirmed tumor	2
Radiolocalization on MAb scan was only positive presurgical finding; patient found to have tumor in another location	1

images. However, accurate imaging was not sufficient for the assignment of a beneficial or very beneficial patient management rating, as indicated by the no-effect ratings assigned to 41 patients who had either true positive or true negative scans. Thus, ^{111}In-CYT-103 immunoscintigraphy was diagnostically accurate for more than half (55%) the patients in whom it was not considered to contribute to management decisions. Likewise, the detection of occult tumor lesions was not sufficient grounds for beneficial or very beneficial ratings, which were assigned to 9 of 11 patients for whom antibody imaging identified occult disease.

As immunoscintigraphy was only one source of diagnostic information derived from the patients' presurgical workup, it is not surprising that diagnostically accurate antibody scan results did not always translate into beneficial patient management impact. Similarly, false positive and false negative findings were not necessarily associated with negative patient management ratings.

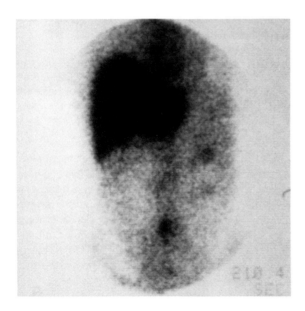

Figure 1 Anterior planar gamma camera images of a patient evaluated for recurrence of ovarian carcinoma. With the exception of antibody imaging, the patient had a negative presurgical workup. The antibody scans identified multiple nodules on the anterior abdominal wall and in the pelvis; these findings were subsequently confirmed at second-look surgery.

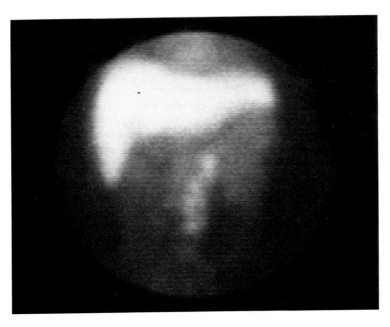

Figure 2 Anterior planar gamma camera images of a patient evaluated prior to second-look laparotomy. Prior to antibody imaging, the patient's presurgical workup demonstrated no evidence of residual disease. Antibody imaging showed radiolocalization in the periaortic lymph node area, which correlated with the tumor detected at surgery.

An examination of the antibody imaging results for the patients assigned ratings of beneficial or very beneficial helps to delineate the performance characteristics associated with positive contributions to the patients' management (Table 4). As shown, immunoscintigraphy was considered to have a beneficial effect on the management of patients in cases where it provided new or unique diagnostic information, including the detection of previously occult lesions. In general, the accurate identification of miliary or microscopic lesions in the abdomen or pelvis as well as lymph node metastases was considered to positively contribute to patient management decisions. Figures 1 and 2 illustrate two cases in which the detection of miliary disease and lymph node metastases, respectively, by antibody imaging was considered to have a beneficial effect on patient management. In some cases, the mere confirmation of such lesions was rated as beneficial or very beneficial. Beneficial ratings were also assigned in cases where the antibody scans correctly suggested a benign etiology for patients with undiagnosed pelvic masses.

DISCUSSION

The results of this multicenter trial confirmed the findings of our preliminary clinical study [20] and demonstrate the utility of ^{111}In-CYT-103 immunoscintigraphy as a diagnostic and staging modality for patients with ovarian carcinoma. The sensitivity of antibody imaging, which is discussed in detail in Chapter 7 is comparable to or better than that of other available diagnostic tests for this disease [5,6,9]. Furthermore, the assessments of the clinical investigators who conducted this trial demonstrate that the results of ^{111}In-CYT-103 immunoscintigraphy have the potential to contribute to the medical and surgical management of certain patients with ovarian cancer.

The results of these assessments also indicate that diagnostic accuracy is not always synonymous with a beneficial impact on patient management. Conversely, inaccurate findings do not necessarily result in a detrimental effect. In general, the antibody scan results associated with positive patient management effects are those that identified occult tumor lesions, specifically miliary or microscopic tumor deposits and lymph node metastases; confirmed the findings of other diagnostic tests and, therefore, increased the physician's confidence that an appropriate surgical procedure would be undertaken; or assisted in the correct assignment of a benign or malignant etiology to an undiagnosed pelvic mass. These results indicate that patient benefit is likely in cases where antibody imaging provided new or confirmatory data to supplement the other evaluations that comprised the presurgical workup.

The ability of antibody imaging to detect carcinomatosis, often consisting of small peritoneal or serosal implants, is an important finding. Diffuse miliary disease is quite common in advanced ovarian carcinoma, and other diagnostic tests are limited in their ability to detect these tumor deposits. In one series of 48 ovarian cancer patients who underwent second-look laparotomy, 52% of those with residual or recurrent disease had carcinomatosis; in 23% of this group, miliary lesions were the only disease detected at surgery [23].

The detection of carcinomatosis by antibody imaging can be beneficial for the management of patients with suspected primary ovarian carcinoma as well as for chemotherapy-treated patients prior to second-look laparotomy. In the former instance, an accurate presurgical assessment of disease will facilitate accurate initial surgical staging and effective debulking, which will, in turn, contribute to the optimal selection of postsurgical therapy and improve the patient's response to subsequent adjuvant treatment. In patients evaluated for residual disease after the completion of first-line chemotherapy, the detection of diffuse, subclinical disease could contribute to a decision to perform a more limited operative procedure (e.g., laparoscopy) or to cancel or delay second-look surgical procedures and to administer additional courses of chemotherapy.

In the present study, false positive antibody scans were considered to have had a negative impact on the management of two patients who were found to be free of malignant disease at surgery. However, false positive antibody images were rated as having no effect on the management of 11 other patients. As with other diagnostic imaging tests, antibody imaging should not be utilized in isolation to make decisions concerning patient management. The results of the antibody scan interpretations should be reviewed in conjunction with information obtained from other diagnostic evaluations in order to establish the optimal patient management plan. When used in this context, immunoscintigraphy with ^{111}In-CYT-103 can provide diagnostic information that can aid in the medical/surgical management of a significant number of patients evaluated for either primary or recurrent ovarian carcinoma.

ACKNOWLEDGMENTS

Appreciation is expressed to the following principal clinical investigators who, in addition to the author, participated in the ^{111}In-CYT-103 multicenter clinical trial: J. Gale Katterhagen, M.D. (Memorial Cancer Center, Springfield, Il); Jon A. Kotler, M.D. (Cleveland Clinic, Florida); Edith P. Mitchell, M.D. (University of Missouri); Ruth Oratz, M.D. (New York University Medical Center); Larry J. Copeland, M.D. (Ohio State University); William J. Mann, M.D. (State University of New York at Stony Brook); Holly H. Gallion, M.D. (University of Kentucky); Donald G. Gallup, M.D. (Medical College of Georgia); David N. Krag, M.D. (University of California at Davis); Gary Purnell, M.D. (University of Arkansas for Medical Sciences); Gregorio Delgado, M.D. (Georgetown University Hospital); Aldo N. Serafini, M.D. (University of Miami School of Medicine); Edgardo L. Yordan, Jr., M.D. (Rush–Presbyterian–St. Luke's Medical Center, Illinois); Bruce R. Line, M.D., and John H. Malfetano, M.D. (Albany Medical College, New York); George Q. Mills, M.D. (Our Lady of the Lake Regional Medical Center, Louisiana); Howard D. Homesley, M.D. (Bowman Gray School of Medicine, North Carolina); and W. Newlon Tauxe, M.D., and Geoffrey Levine, Ph.D. (Presbyterian–University Hospital, Pittsburgh, Pennsylvania). This multicenter study was supported by a grant from CYTOGEN Corporation (Princeton, NJ).

REFERENCES

1.   American Cancer Society. Cancer facts and figures. Atlanta, GA:American Cancer Society, 1989:11.
2.   Disaia PJ, Creasman WT. Clinical gynecologic oncology. St. Louis: Mosby, 1989:292–416.

3. Young RC. Gynecologic cancers. In:Wittes RE, ed. Manual of Oncologic herapeutics. Philadelphia: Lippincott, 1989:270-6.
4. Fisher RI, Young RC. Chemotherapy of ovarian cancer. Surg Clin North Am 1978; 58:143.
5. Young RC, Fuks Z, Hoskins WJ. Cancer of the ovary. In:DeVita VT, JR, Hellman S, Rosenberg SA, eds. Cancer Principles and Practices of Oncology. Philadelphia:Lippincott, 1989:1162-96.
6. Smith LH, Oi RH. Detection of malignant ovarian neoplasms: a review of the literature. I. Detection of the patient at risk: clinical, radiological, and cytological detection. Obstet Gynecol Surv 1984; 39:313-28.
7. McGowan L, Parent Lesher L, Norris HL, Barnett M. Misstaging of ovarian cancer. Obstet Gynecol 1985; 65:568-72.
8. Piver MS. Ovarian carcinoma: a decade of progress. Cancer 1984; 54:2706-15.
9. Ozols RF, Young RC. Ovarian cancer. Curr Probl Cancer 1987; 11:57-122.
10. Sonnendecker EWW. Is routine second-look laparotomy for ovarian cancer justified? Gynecol Oncol 1988; 31:249-55.
11. Haller DG. Monoclonal antibody imaging in the management of patients with colorectal cancer. J Clin Oncol 1988; 6:1213-5.
12. Larson SM. Lymphoma, melanoma, colon cancer: diagnosis and treatment with radiolabeled monoclonal antibodies. Radiology 1987; 165:297-304.
13. Byers VS, Baldwin RW. Therapeutic strategies with monoclonal antibodies and immunoconjugates. Immunology 1988; 65:329-35.
14. Shepherd JH, Granowska M, Britton FE, et al. Tumor-associated monoclonal antibodies for diagnosis and assessment of ovarian cancer. Br J Obstet Gynecol 1987; 94:160-7.
15. Pateisky N, Philipp K, Skodler WD, Czerwenka K, Hamilton G, Burchell J. Radioimmunodetection in patients with suspected ovarian cancer. J Nucl Med 1985; 26:1369-76.
16. Granowska M, Shepherd J, Britton KE, et al. Ovarian cancer: diagnosis using ^{123}I monoclonal antibody in comparison with surgical findings. Nucl Med Commun 1984; 5:485-99.
17. Hunter RE, Doherty P, Griffen TW, et al. Use of indium-111 labeled OC-125 monoclonal antibody in the detection of ovarian cancer. Gynecol Oncol 1987; 27:325-37.
18. Simpson J, Schlom J. The use of monoclonal antibody B72.3 in the management of gynecologic malignancies. Yale J Biol Med 1988; 61:351-66.
19. Mansi L, Panza N, Lastoria S, Pacilio G, Salvatore M. Diagnosis of ovarian cancer with radiolabeled monoclonal antibodies: our experience using ^{131}I-B72.3. Nucl Med Biol 1989; 16:127-35.
20. Surwit E, and the OncoScint OV103 Multicenter Study Group. Use of a radiolabeled immunoconjugate of MAb B72.3 (^{111}In-CYT-103, OncoScint OV103) for the detection of epithelial ovarian carcinoma. Antibody Immunoconjugates Radiopharmaceut 1990; 3:44.
21. Schlom J, Colcher D, Roselli M, et al. Tumor targeting with monoclonal antibody B72.3. Nucl Med Biol 1989; 16:137-42.

22. Rodwell JD, Alvarez VL, Lee C, et al. Site-specific covalent modification of monoclonal antibodies: in vitro and in vivo evaluations. Proc Natl Acad Sci USA 1986; 83:2632–6.

23. Silverman PM, Osbourne M, Dunnick NR, Bandy LC. CT prior to second-look operation in ovarian cancer. Am J Roentgenol 1988; 150:829–32.

9

Oncoscint Image Atlas

Robert T. Maguire
CYTOGEN Corporation, Princeton, New Jersey

The purpose of this chapter is to familiarize the reader with the pattern of OncoScint uptake in patients with colorectal or ovarian malignancies. In addition, the distribution of this reagent in patients without disease or in those with various benign disorders is also demonstrated. OncoScint is a whole body imaging agent and may be utilized as a "road map" to direct confirmatory anatomical imaging modalities such as computed tomography (CT) or magnetic resonance imaging (MRI), and to aid the surgeon in the preoperative decision-making process.

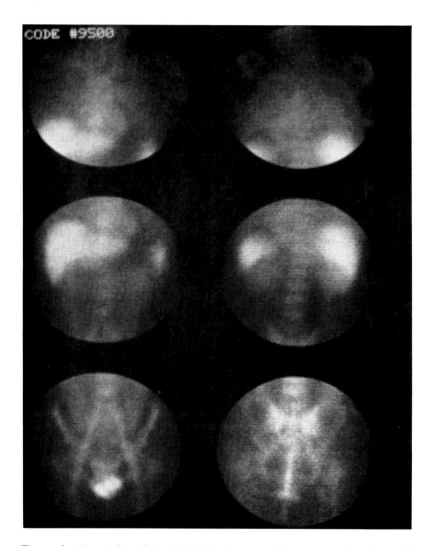

Figure 1 Normal OncoScint biodistribution. Anterior and posterior views of the thorax, abdomen, and pelvis taken at 48 and 72 hr in a 40-year-old male without evidence of malignancy upon surgical exploration. Blood pool activity is demonstrated in the heart and major vessels. Bone marrow activity appears by 24 hr and remains present throughout the study. Liver and spleen activity appear shortly following injection and remain present throughout the study. The distribution of activity within these organs should be relatively uniform with both organs having normal size and

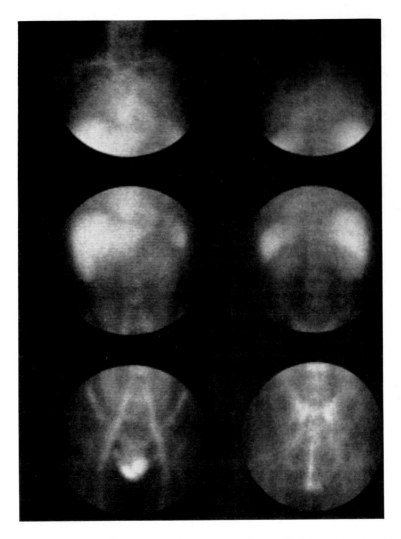

shape. Faint renal uptake may be present as late as 3–4 days following injection. Intense images of the rectal area which is thought to represent the buttocks crease. Though not apparent in this set of images, urinary bladder activity can be seen in some patients. Generally, this activity is more apparent on anterior views, whereas pelvic tumor masses are more intense on posterior views. (A) 48 hr anterior, (B) 48 hr posterior, (C) 72 hr anterior, (D) 72 hr posterior.

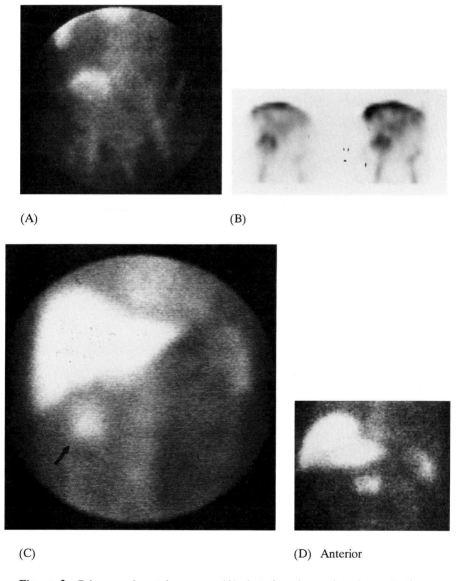

(A)   (B)

(C)   (D) Anterior

Figure 2   Primary colorectal cancer. (A) Anterior planar view demonstrating localization to the right lower quadrant in the area of a surgically confirmed cecal tumor. (B) Coronal SPECT view demonstrating more avid uptake in the periphery of this large tumor. (C) Hepatic flexure adenocarcinoma (arrow). (D) Transverse

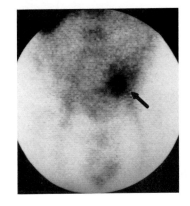

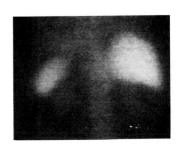

(D) Posterior   (E)

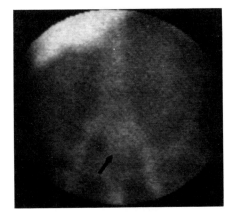

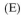

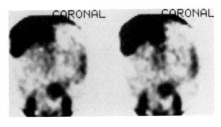

(F) Anterior Planar View   (F) Coronal SPECT Images

colon adenocarcinoma. Note increased localization on anterior versus posterior abdominal view. (E) Anterior pelvic view demonstrating primary sigmoid carcinoma with local extension. (F) Patient with surgically confirmed sigmoid carcinoma. Anterior planar view suggestive of large lesion, which is confirmed by coronal SPECT images.

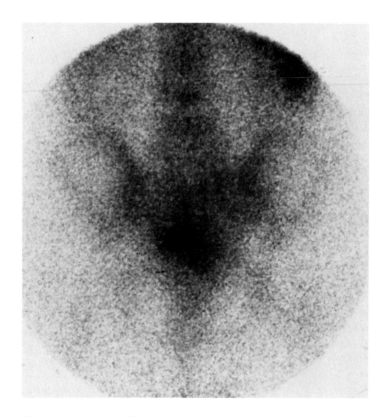

(G) Posterior Pelvic View

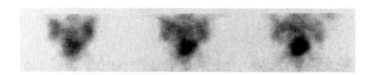

(G) Coronal SPECT Image

Figure 2 Continued

(G) Posterior whole body and pelvic views of patient with primary rectal carcinoma. Large tumor is well demonstrated on coronal SPECT images.

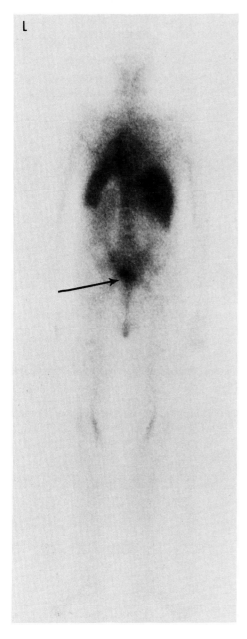

(G) Whole body view

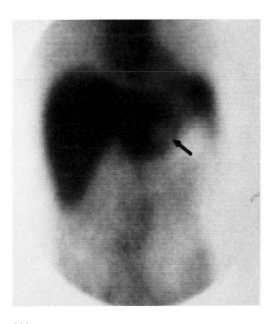

(A)

Figure 3 Patterns of hepatic metastases. (A) Isolated hepatic recurrence – Patients with isolated hepatic recurrences from colorectal cancer are potentially candidates for curative resection. Hepatic lesions generally appear as photopenic defects on OncoScint images (arrow). (B) Generalized hepatic involvement. (C) SPECT imaging of the liver — in this patient, hepatic SPECT views readily demonstrated a metastatic lesion (arrow) which was not obvious on planar views. Lesion was confirmed at surgery.

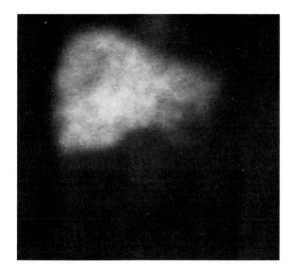

(B)

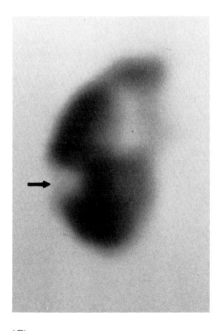

(C)

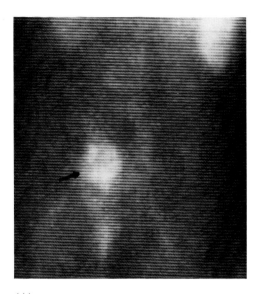

(A)

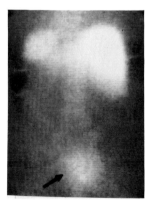

(B)

Figure 4 Isolated pelvic recurrence. (A,B) Planar scintigraphs of two patients with isolated and potentially resectable pelvic recurrences. Such lesions are more readily apparent on posterior views.

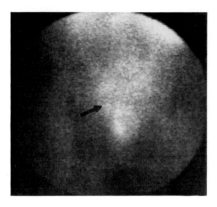

(C)

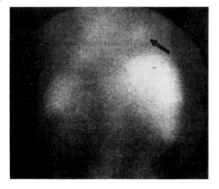

(D)

(C and D) Patient initially thought to have an isolated pelvic recurrence (C), who had a left lung metastasis detected on posterior planar OncoScint image (D). The previously scheduled surgical procedure was canceled.

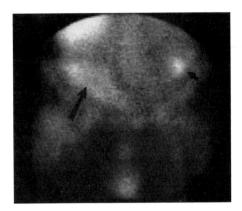

Figure 5 Metachronous recurrence. Anterior planar view of pelvis demonstrating localization to a surgically confirmed cecal adenocarcinoma (long arrow) in a patient who had undergone previous resection of his sigmoid carcinoma. Colostomy site (short arrow) is evident in left mid-abdomen.

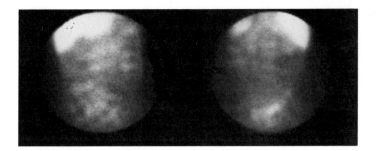

Figure 6　Carcinomatosis.　Patient with suspected local recurrence in the area of her previously resected ascending colon primary with widespread intraperitoneal disease demonstrated on OncoScint scans.

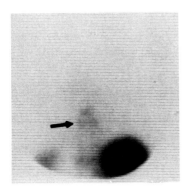

(A)

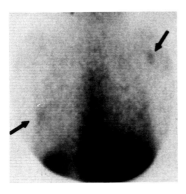

(B)

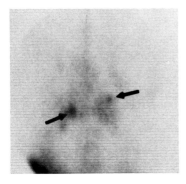

(C)

Figure 7 Patterns of bony metastases. (A,B,C). This patient with known primary colorectal cancer and liver metastases had multiple areas of bone involvement noted on OncoScint scan, including lesions of the thoracic spine (A), right shoulder and left seventh rib (B), and right and left pelvis (C). These lesions were confirmed by bone scan and the rib lesion was confirmed by a biopsy procedure. The previously planned hepatic artery catheter placement was canceled.

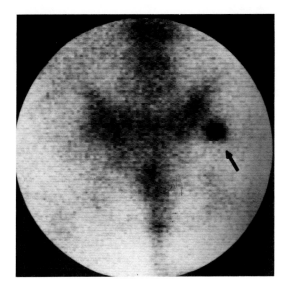

(D)

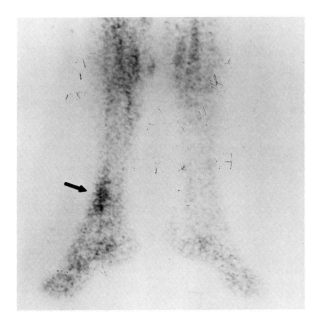

(E)

(D) Patient with a known primary lesion of the rectum with OncoScint localization to an unsuspected bone lesion in the right iliac bone. (E) Posterior OncoScint image demonstrating a biopsy-confirmed metastatic lesion of the left ankle in a patient with primary malignancy of the descending colon.

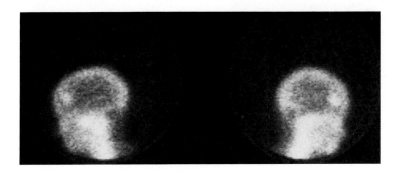

(A)

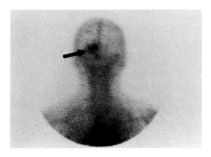

(B)

Figure 8 Patterns of recurrence — brain metastases. (A) Patient with recurrent abdominal tumor and bone metastases with occult brain metastasis detected by OncoScint scan. (B) Patient with previously irradiated colorectal cancer brain metastasis and rising CEA. OncoScint scan demonstrates active brain metastasis.

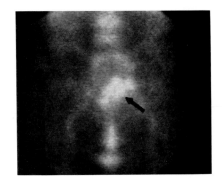

(A)

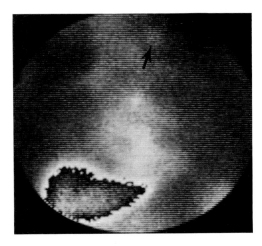

(B)

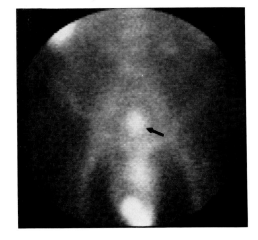

(C)

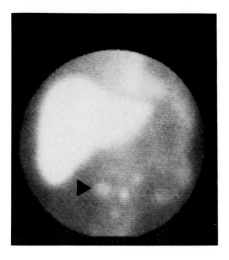

(D)

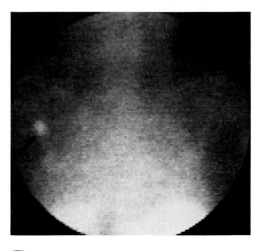

(E)

Figure 9 Patterns of recurrence — miscellaneous cases. (A) Repeat OncoScint scan demonstrating a recurrent pelvic mass in an area of previous colorectal cancer surgery. (B) Demonstration of previously undetected metastasis in a lymph node in the neck of a patient with surgically confirmed carcinoma of the cecum. The ability of OncoScint scans to view the entire body allows this modality to function as a road map for subsequent confirmatory diagnostic procedures. (C,D,E) Patient with a known recurrent pelvic lesion (C), with demonstration of additional mid-abdominal lesions (D), and a scapular lesion (E), subsequently documented on bone scan.

ONCOSCINT OVARIAN CANCER IMAGES

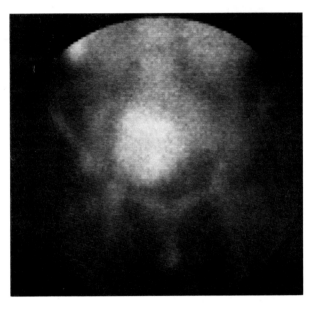

(A)

Figure 10 Primary ovarian cancers. (A) Anterior planar view of a 76-year-old woman with primary serous papillary carcinoma of the right ovary. (B) Stage III endometrioid carcinoma of the right ovary with extensive tumor involvement of the anterior abdominal wall. (C) Anterior and posterior planar views of the pelvis in a 50-year-old female with primary papillary serous carcinoma involving both ovaries, omentum, and regional lymph nodes. Note the hazy appearance of the abdomen on the anterior view. Approximately 1 L of ascites was present.

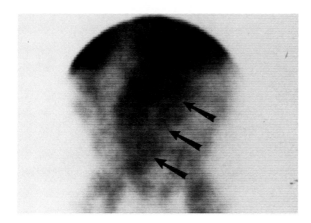

(B)

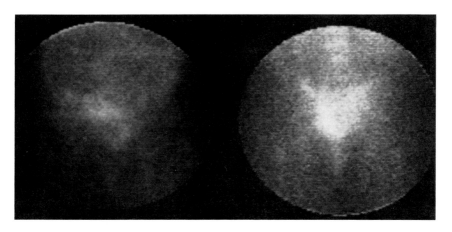

(C) Anterior   Posterior

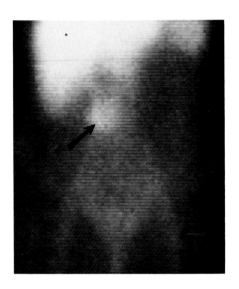

(A) Anterior

Figure 11 Ovarian carcinoma — patterns of recurrence. (A) Patient with stage III ovarian carcinoma after completion of platinum-based chemotherapy. Anterior planar OncoScint scan reveals the presence of a large paraaortic lymph node which was confirmed as the site of tumor recurrence at surgery. (B) Patient with stage III carcinoma of the ovary status post–platinum-based chemotherapy. Anterior and posterior OncoScint scans demonstrate anterior abdominal wall and pelvic recurrences, which were confirmed at surgery. (C) Patient with stage III carcinoma of the ovary after chemotherapy. OncoScint scan localized to surgically confirmed disease in the anterior abdominal wall and pelvis. (D) Anterior and posterior planar OncoScint scans revealing recurrent pelvic mass and widespread carcinomatosis involving the anterior abdomen. (E) Additional example of carcinomatosis in a patient 6 months after completion of chemotherapy for stage III ovarian carcinoma. CT scan findings were equivocal. The OncoScint scan localized to multiple surgically confirmed sites within the abdomen and pelvis. (F) A 65-year-old female patient with stage III ovarian carcinoma, who received chemotherapy and had a negative second-look operative procedure. She then developed a gradually rising CA-125 level and an inguinal mass. The OncoScint scan localized well to this lesion, which was surgically confirmed as recurrent ovarian carcinoma. (G) A 44-year-old female patient 2 years after chemotherapy for stage III ovarian carcinoma. She had a mildly elevated CA-125 level and a negative CT scan of the abdomen. OncoScint scan revealed paraaortic lymphadenopathy, which was the only site of tumor recurrence noted at surgery.

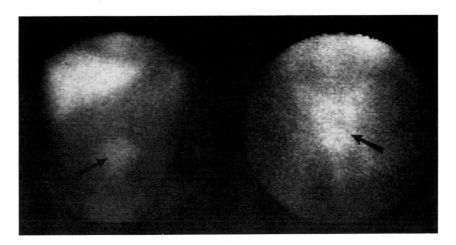

(B) Posterior

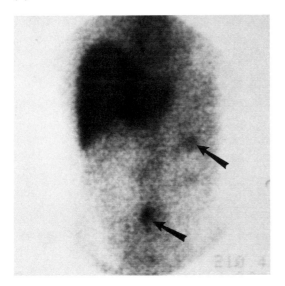

(C) Anterior

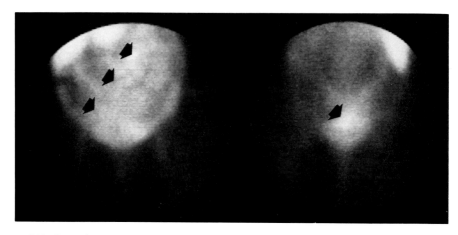

(D) Posterior

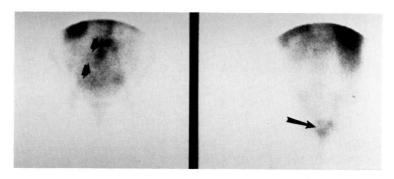

(E) Anterior   Posterior

Figure 11 Continued

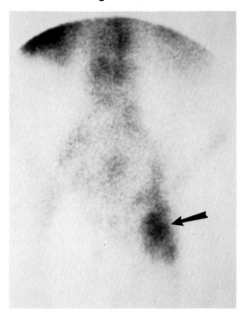

(F)

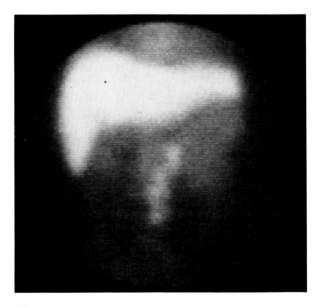

(G)

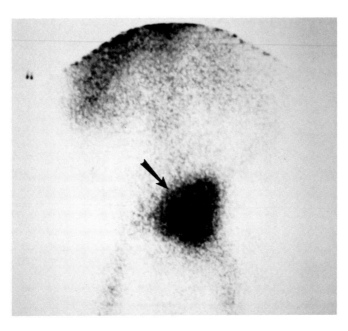

(A)

Figure 12 Benign ovarian lesions (A) Large ovarian fibroma. Occasional benign ovarian tumors may express the TAG-72 antigen. (B) A 74-year-old female with an ovarian fibroma and a large simple serous cyst. (C) Anterior planar pelvic view of a 46-year-old female with a large pelvic mass determined to be a hemorrhagic, cystic corpus luteum originating in the left ovary.

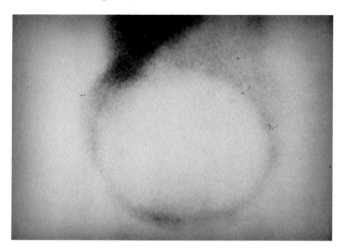

(B)

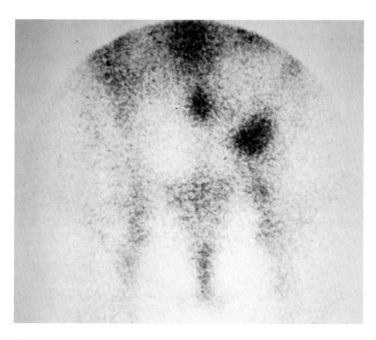

(C)

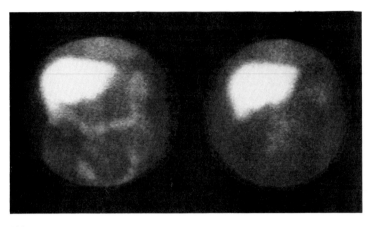

(A)

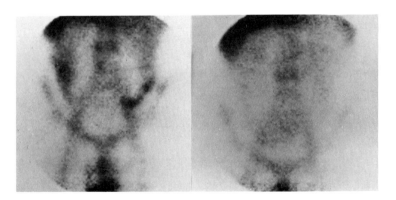

(B)

Figure 13 Nonspecific bowel patterns. (A,B) Images of two patients at 48 and 72 hr demonstrating pronounced stool uptake on initial images with clearing by the time of the second imaging session. Cathartics may be useful between imaging sessions in patients with suspected localization in stool.

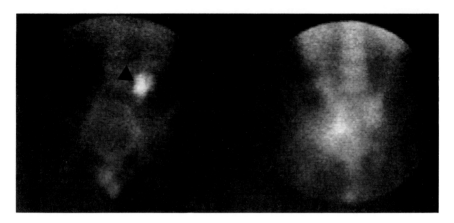

(A) Anterior

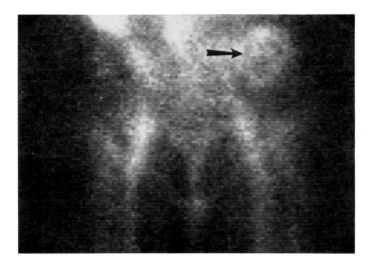

(B) Posterior

Figure 14 Colostomy sites. (A,B) Localization to colostomy sites (arrows) in (A) a patient with a confirmed pelvic recurrence on the posterior view, and (B) a patient 1.5 years after colorectal cancer resection. OncoScint localization in normal colostomy sites is a common finding.

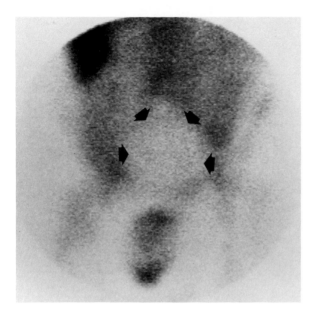

Figure 15 Urinary bladder. Photopenic area representing urinary bladder is clearly demonstrated on this anterior OncoScint image. Occasionally, the urinary bladder contains increased OncoScint activity.

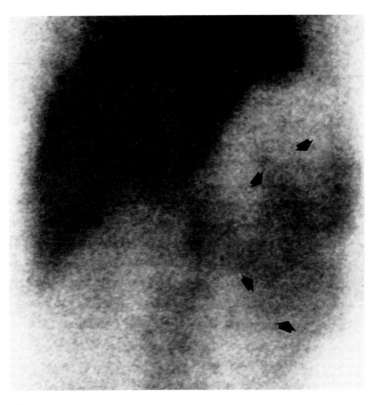

(A)

Figure 16 Areas of inflammation. (A,B) Areas of inflammation may be localized by OncoScint scans as demonstrated in an individual with a surgically confirmed pericolic area of inflammation after a colonoscopic biopsy procedure (A), and in an individual with arthritis of the right shoulder and a history of a recent fracture in this area (B).

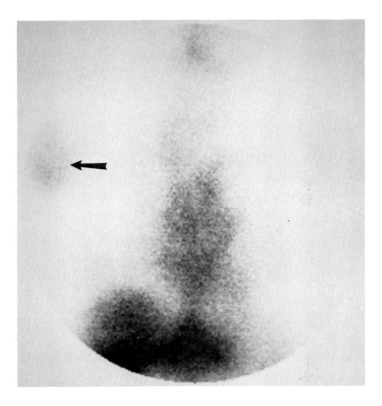

(B)

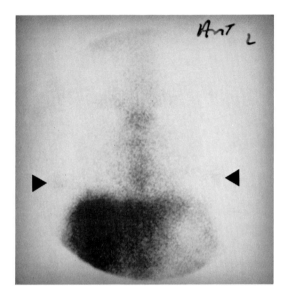

Figure 17 Breast nipple shadows. Occasionally, breast nipple shadows are noted in females receiving OncoScint. The location and symmetry of this finding makes the image interpretation fairly straightforward. It should be noted, however, that OncoScint may also localize to primary carcinomas in the breast.

10

Immunopharmacokinetics of ^{111}In-CYT-103 in Ovarian Cancer Patients

William J. Jusko and Li-Pin Kung
State University of New York at Buffalo, Buffalo, New York

Raymond F. Schmelter
CYTOGEN Corporation, Princeton, New Jersey

INTRODUCTION

Murine monoclonal antibodies (MAb) which have been physically modified by labeling with either gamma- or particle- emitting radionuclides are increasingly being used for diagnosis or therapy of life-threatening diseases. For example, whole IgG antibodies directed against tumor-associated antigens have been radiolabeled with either ^{111}In, ^{131}I, or ^{99m}Tc for the diagnostic imaging of a variety of malignancies. Similarly, whole IgG antibodies labeled with either ^{90}Y or ^{131}I are the subject of several current clinical investigations as potential therapeutic agents.

MAb B72.3, which was developed by Schlom and co-workers [1–3], has undergone intensive study because of its wide pattern of reactivity with a variety of mucin-producing adenocarcinomas and limited reactivity with normal tissues. MAb B72.3 is an IgG_1 antibody that targets a high-molecular-weight ($>10^6$ Dalton) [4], tumor-associated glycoprotein called TAG-72. The TAG-72 antigen is expressed on the surface of certain human colon, breast, and ovarian carcinoma cell lines. This ability of antibody B72.3 to bind adenocarcinomas was incorporated into a multicenter clinical trial in which the murine monoclonal served as a targeting vehicle to localize ^{111}In for imaging of patients with ovarian carcinoma. The murine antibody molecule was modified by site-specifically conjugating it with the linker-chelator glycine-tyrosine-(N-ϵ-DTPA)-lysine [5] and radiolabeling it with [111]In. The radiolabeled antibody conjugate was intravenously injected into 103 patients with known or suspected primary or recurrent/ residual ovarian carcinoma. This chapter describes the pharmacokinetics in a subset of that population.

METHODS

Patients

Pharmacokinetic data were assessed for 26 women enrolled at three study sites. The women ranged in age from 34 to 83 years and had not received antitumor therapy for 4 weeks prior to MAb infusion. The clinical characteristics of the individual patients are listed in Table 1.

Antibody Administration

One-milligram doses of the MAb conjugate were radiolabeled with 4.1-5.7mCi ^{111}In chloride (Amersham) according to a standard procedure. The radiochemical purity of the ^{111}In-chelated antibody was verified by instant thin-layer chromatography (ITLC-SG) and found to be $\geq 95\%$. The radiolabeled MAb conjugate was infused intravenously over 5–10 min.

Sampling Procedures

Serial blood samples were taken prior to infusion and at 5, 15, 30, 60, 90, 120, and 240 min after infusion. Additional samples were obtained between 2 and 7 days postinfusion. Urine was collected after dosing over the following time periods: 0–2 hr, 2–24 hr, and then at 24-hr intervals up to 7 days postinfusion.

Assays

Duplicate 1-ml aliquots of plasma or urine were counted in a gamma-ray scintillation counter adjusted for an ^{111}In energy window. Standards prepared from an aliquot of the administered ^{111}In-CYT-103 dose were counted at the same time to correct for radioactive decay.

Pharmacokinetic Analysis

Plasma ^{111}In-CYT-103 concentrations (Cp) or radioactivity (CPM) as a function of time (t) was characterized by either a monoexponential equation:

$$C_p = C_o \cdot e^{-k \cdot t} \tag{1}$$

or a biexponential equation:

$$C_p = C_1 \cdot e^{-\ \cdot t} + C_2 \cdot e^{-\ _2 \cdot t} \tag{2}$$

Table 1 Clinical Characteristics of Study Patients

Pt. no.	Age (yr)	Ht (in.)	Wt (lb)	Creatine in (mg/dl)	BUN (mg/dl)	SGOT (U/L)	Alk. phos. (U/L)	Bili-rubin (mg/dl)	Other drugs Beta-blockers	Premarin
105-1	61	65.75	149	1.0	18	29	115	0.4	-	-
105-2	72	64	116	1.3	22	41	55	0.3	+	-
105-3	66	61.25	168	1.1	27	31	69	0.4	-	+
105-4	68	61	178	1.6	34	38	141	0.5	+	-
105-5	55	65	140	1.2	24	37	48	0.4	-	+
105-6	59	65	182	1.2	24	37	70	0.3	-	+
105-7	67	63	138	1.2	28	16	72	0.4	-	+
105-8	34	65	118	0.8	13	18	46	0.4	-	+
105-9	57	70	173	0.9	11	14	109	0.9	-	-
105-10	50	67	159	1.3	19	31	48	0.3	-	-
105-11	55	68	227	1.6	41	20	67	0.4	+	-
105-12	50	61	117	0.7	4	51	75	0.5	-	-
105-13	62	62.5	112	1.0	16	21	122	0.4	-	-
105-14	34	62.5	123	0.8	14	17	38	0.6	-	-
105-15	60	67	197	1.8	25	17	43	0.3	-	-
105-16	73	62	97	0.5	19	24	22	0.7	-	-
105-17	52	64	125	1.2	19	22	23	0.5	-	+
105-18	72	ND	117	1.0	20	47	31	0.9	+	-
105-19	53	65	137	1.3	18	22	52	0.4	-	+
155-1	71	ND	ND	0.9	9	28	59	0.4	-	-
155-2	54	65	139	0.9	14	15	68	0.2	-	-
155-3	77	64.5	163	0.7	6	26	149	0.1	-	-
155-4	71	66	175	0.9	13	65	177	2.4	+	-
155-5	70	59	125	1.6	44	10	81	0.4	-	-
186-1	83	64	129	0.9	13	34	58	0.3	-	-
186-2	46	63	195	0.7	16	13	80	0.7	-	-

ND, not determined.

in order to generate the intercepts Cp or C_1 and C_2 and disposition slopes (k or $_1$ and $_2$). Because the infusion time was brief compared to the disposition half-life, the plasma data were treated as an intravenous bolus administration. Least-squares fitting was performed using the NONLIN computer program [6]. Clearance (CL) was then calculated from dose/AUC (area under the plasma concentration curve), where AUC was obtained from C_o/k for the monoexponential data or from $C_1/_1 = C_2/_2$ for the biexponential data. Volume of distribution (V or V_{ss} was obtained as the ratio of dose and initial plasma concentration (C_o) for monoexponential cases and from CL · MRT for biexponential cases where: MRT = $(C_1/_1^2 + C_2/_2^2)$/AUC [7]. The elimination half-life ($t_{1/2}$) was obtained from either 0.693/k (monoexponential) or from 0.693/$_2$ (biexponential).

Apparent renal clearance was obtained from:

$$CL_R = Ae_{(t1 - t2)}/AUC_{(t1 - t2)} \tag{3}$$

in which $Ae_{(t1 - t2)}$ is the amount of radioactivity in urine collected from $t1$ to $t2$; $t1$ and $t2$ are the times for the beginning and the end of the urine collection during the study; and $AUC_{(t1 - t2)}$ is the area under the plasma concentration of ^{111}In-CYT-103 from $t1$ to $t2$. The AUC $_{(t1 - t2)}$ was determined either from (monoexponential):

$$AUC_{(t1 - t2)} = (C_o/k) \cdot e^{-k \cdot t1} - (C_o/k) \cdot e^{-k \cdot t2} \tag{4}$$

or from (biexponential):

$$AUC_{(t1 - t2)} =$$
$$(C_1/_1)(e^{-_1 \cdot t1} - e^{-_1 \cdot t2}) + (C_2/_2)(e^{-_2 \cdot t1} - e^{-_2 \cdot t2}) \tag{5}$$

Clearance and volume of distribution were normalized by ideal body weight (IBW), which was estimated from height for females by the formula [8]:

$$IBW \ (kg) = 45 \pm 2.3 \ \text{per inch above or below 5 ft.} \tag{6}$$

Creatinine clearance was estimated from serum creatinine concentration (S_{cr}) for females by Cockcroft and Gault [9]:

$$CL_{CR} \ (ml/min) = 0.85 \cdot (140 - age) \cdot (weight/72)/S_{CR} \tag{7}$$

The data are presented as the mean ± standard deviation. Statistical evaluations utilized Student's t test. The Akaike Information Criterion (AIC) was employed to help discriminate between the mono- and biexponential curve fittings as optimal for each patient's disposition profile [10].

RESULTS

Patient Data

Plasma data were obtained from 26 patients and urinary data from 20 patients. The disposition data tended to emphasize the early time period and relatively few samples were collected beyond 5 hr. This sometimes caused difficulty in characterizing the elimination phase when using the biexponential equation. Thus data from all patients were initially fitted with the monoexponential function (Eq. 1).

Pharmacokinetics

Typical plots of percentage of injected dose per liter of plasma versus time are shown for two patients in Figure 1. Concentration-time profiles for the ovarian cancer patients studied yielded a monoexponential decline with a half-life of 50 ± 14 hr, while nine patients showed a biexponential decline with an elimination half-life of 62 ± 12 hr.

Monoexponential parameters estimated from the plasma data for all patients are presented in Table 2; biexponential parameters are provided for nine patients in Table 3. Clearances and volumes of distribution listed in Table 4 were based on the optimum fitting of the exponential data (as indicated). Patient 186-2 appeared to be an outlier with extremely high CL and V values and was not included in the further analyses and data presentation. The general $t_{\frac{1}{2}}$ of the group averaged 56 ± 14 hr. The plasma clearance of ^{111}In-CYT-103 averaged 50 ± 15 (range: 25 to 81) ml/hr, the volume of distribution averaged 3.8 ± 1.2 liters, and apparent renal clearance averaged 4.9 ± 2.1 ml/hr. Only a small fraction ($CL_r/CL = 10\%$) of the administered radioactivity was excreted in urine over 72 hr.

Several pathophysiological factors that often affect xenobiotic disposition were assessed. The degree of obesity was expressed as the ratio: total body weight (TBW)/ideal body weight (IBW). As shown in Figure 2, CL and V are essentially constant with the TBW/IBW ratios; therefore, these parameters were normalized by ideal body weight (see Table 4 for normalized data). Patient ages spanned 34–83 years. Figure 3 shows that normalized CL and V are independent of age.

Creatinine clearance (CL_{CR}) and bilirubin concentrations are commonly used clinical markers for renal and hepatic function. Normalized CL did not correlate with either of these factors in this group (Fig. 4).

An evaluation was also made to determine whether the use (see Table 1) of either beta-blockers or Premarin (Wyeth-Ayerst) affected the CL of ^{111}In-CYT-103. Estrogens often inhibit hepatic metabolism. Neither beta-blockers ($CL_{with} = 1.037 ± 0.508$; $CL_{without} = 0.992 ± 0.332$) nor Premarin ($CL_{with} = 0.912 ± 0.098$; $CL_{without} = 0.992 ± 0.332$) was a significant factor.

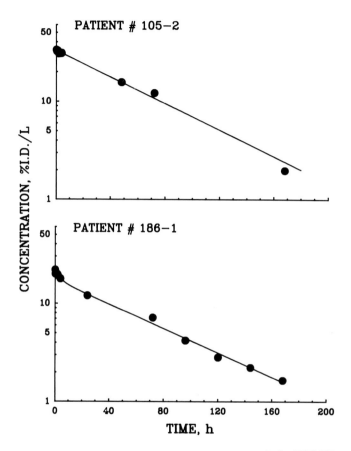

Figure 1 Typical profiles of plasma concentrations of ^{111}In-CYT-103 as percent injected dose per liter (%ID/L) versus time in two patients.

Table 2 Pharmacokinetic Parameters of ^{111}In-CYT-103 Using Monoexponential Fitting

Pt. no.	C_o (%ID/L)	k (1/hr)	$t\frac{1}{2}$ (hr)	r^2	AIC
105-1	49.17 ± 1.29[a]	0.02488 ± 0.00248	27.9	0.965	28.89
105-2	32.76 ± 0.45	0.01550 ± 0.00053	44.7	0.997	17.54
105-3	26.90 ± 0.79	0.01260 ± 0.00141	55.0	0.932	32.11
105-4	24.61 ± 0.82	0.02006 ± 0.00147	34.5	0.989	24.57
105-5	26.60 ± 0.31	0.01333 ± 0.00050	52.0	0.996	11.66
105-6	20.90 ± 0.10	0.01171 ± 0.00022	59.2	0.998	-5.57
105-7	17.61 ± 0.69	0.00882 ± 0.00161	78.6	0.856	25.02
105-8	27.59 ± 0.30	0.01614 ± 0.00054	42.9	0.995	9.99
105-9	27.16 ± 0.47	0.01525 ± 0.00075	45.4	0.989	20.57
105-10	21.48 ± 0.21	0.01425 ± 0.00046	48.6	0.995	4.73
105-11	15.52 ± 0.08	0.01025 ± 0.00035	67.6	0.993	-8.79
105-12	30.80 ± 1.35	0.01220 ± 0.00311	56.8	0.782	30.51
105-13	20.49 ± 0.43	0.01021 ± 0.00053	67.9	0.994	4.35
105-14	27.70 ± 0.63	0.01179 ± 0.00086	58.8	0.988	13.28
105-15	27.21 ± 0.43	0.01538 ± 0.00082	45.1	0.985	20.42
105-16	NA	0.01311 ± 0.00077	52.8	0.981	0.14
105-17	NA	0.01327 ± 0.00056	52.2	0.993	13.86
105-18	NA	0.05216 ± 0.00387	13.3	0.998	10.65
105-19	20.34 ± 0.43	0.00884 ± 0.00090	78.4	0.937	21.79
155-1	46.63 ± 0.87	0.01694 ± 0.00084	40.9	0.995	34.62
155-2	45.88 ± 0.59	0.01667 ± 0.00055	41.6	0.995	27.80
155-3	36.96 ± 1.41	0.01277 ± 0.00095	54.3	0.973	42.59
155-4	41.48 ± 0.51	0.01245 ± 0.00037	55.7	0.995	28.61
155-5	49.32 ± 0.40	0.01568 ± 0.00031	44.2	0.998	13.80
186-1	19.94 ± 0.39	0.01570 ± 0.00056	44.1	0.996	20.41
186-2	11.06 ± 0.32	0.01902 ± 0.00115	36.4	0.991	11.49
Mean	29.05	0.01573	50.0		
SD	11.03	0.00823	14.4		

[a]NONLIN-estimated standard deviations
NA, not available

Table 3 Pharmacokinetic Parameters of ^{111}In-CYT-Using Biexponential Fitting

Pt. no.	C_1 (%ID/L)	$_1$ (1/hr)	C_2 (%ID/L)	$_2$ (1/hr)	$t^{1/2}$ (hr)	r^2	AIC
105-5	3.84	0.0844	23.15	0.01189	58.3	0.988	6.76
105-9	8.80	0.1452	19.58	0.01123	61.7	0.998	8.58
105-17	NA	0.0438	NA	0.00727	72.9	0.997	12.88
105-18	NA	0.0908	NA	0.01569	79.3	0.999	8.51
155-1	13.96	0.0522	35.45	0.01248	55.5	0.997	31.29
155-2	15.12	0.0646	31.59	0.01160	59.8	0.999	8.83
155-4	10.28	0.0496	31.75	0.00946	73.3	0.999	18.71
186-1	3.56	0.2275	17.34	0.01425	48.6	0.998	14.14
186-2	2.87	0.1824	8.81	0.01576	44.0	0.996	6.17
Mean	8.35	0.1045	23.95	0.01218	61.5		
SD	5.08	0.0656	9.52	0.00279	11.8		

NA, not available

DISCUSSION

The results of previous studies in which ^{111}In-labeled MAb B72.3 was administered to patients with colorectal cancer have shown that an initially rapid distribution phase was followed by a slow elimination phase. For example, Yokoyama et al. [4] conjugated the MAb with the bifunctional chelator isothiocyanatobenzyl-DTPA, radiolabeled it with 3–5 mCi ^{111}In, and intravenously infused it into colorectal cancer patients with radiographic evidence of metastatic involvement of the liver. They observed a serum beta half-life of the radiolabeled MAb of 63 ± 5 hr and a 72-hr cumulative urinary excretion of ^{111}In of 7.9 ± 1.35%. Also, Harwood et al. studied the biodistribution of 20–mg doses of intravenously injected ^{111}In-CYT-103 in patients with biopsy proven colon adenocarcinoma [11]. Analysis of serial serum samples demonstrated a biexponential elimination of radiolabeled MAb with a terminal phase serum clearance of 64.2 ± 14.2 hr. The 72-hr cumulative urinary excretion in their patients was 13.0 ± 8.7%.

Nine ovarian cancer patients in the present study demonstrated biexponential plasma clearance following intravenous administration of ^{111}In-CYT-103. The average terminal half-life of 56 ± 14 hr was similar to the values previously reported by these earlier investigators for colorectal cancer patients. However, plasma clearance for other patients in the present study could not readily be ascribed to a biexponential decline, and for those cases both monoexponential and biexponential equations were used in curve fitting. Final pharmacokinetic parameters were calculated using the equation, providing

Table 4 Summary of Primary Pharmacokinetic Parameters.

Pt. no.	Equation	CL (ml/hr)	V_{ss} (L)	$t_{\frac{1}{2}}$ (hr)	CL_R (ml/hr)	CL_{IBM} (ml/hr/kg IBW)	V_{IBW} (ml/kg IBW)
105-1	1[a]	50.59	2.034	27.9	9.36	0.6806	27.36
105-2	1	47.30	3.052	44.7	4.38	0.8726	56.32
105-3	1	46.83	3.717	55.0	5.38	0.9781	77.64
105-4	1	81.51	4.063	34.5	3.66	1.7231	85.90
105-5	2[a]	50.12	4.138	58.3	3.03	0.8870	73.24
105-6	1	56.05	4.784	59.2	7.35	0.9919	84.68
105-7	1	50.09	5.680	78.6	1.73	0.9651	109.44
105-8	1	58.51	3.624	42.9	5.21	1.0355	64.15
105-9	2	56.13	4.780	61.7	4.73	0.8254	70.29
105-10	1	66.35	4.655	48.6	4.23	1.0859	76.18
105-11	1	66.09	6.444	67.7	4.94	1.0424	101.64
105-12	1	39.62	3.247	56.8	3.14	0.8376	68.65
105-13	1	49.85	4.881	67.9	5.34	0.9822	96.19
105-14	1	42.56	3.610	58.8	2.97	0.8386	71.14
105-15	1	56.51	3.675	45.1	4.46	0.9249	60.15
105-16	1	NA	NA	52.8	NA	NA	NA
105-17	2	NA	NA	72.9	NA	NA	NA
105-18	2	NA	NA	79.3	NA	NA	NA
105-19	1	43.48	4.160	78.4	5.14	0.7695	87.01
155-1	2	33.07	2.409	55.5	5.94	NA	NA
155-2	2	36.34	2.726	59.8	4.20	0.6431	48.25
155-3	1	34.56	2.706	54.3	7.55	0.6244	48.88
155-4	2	30.01	2.827	73.3	3.73	0.5104	48.08
155-5	1	25.27	2.028	44.2	6.08	0.5918	47.49
186-1	2	81.13	5.624	48.6	8.12	1.4968	103.76
186-2	2	173.93	10.76	44.0	12.95	3.3506	207.37
Mean		55.47	4.158	56.4	5.51	0.9456	77.90
SD		29.61	1.858	13.4	2.65	0.3017	35.72
Mean+		50.09	3.857	56.9	4.86	0.9194	71.74
SD		14.84	1.203	13.5	2.11	0.2822	32.48

[a]1=monoexponential equation.
[b]2=biexponential equation.
[c]Excluding patient 186-2.
NA, not available.

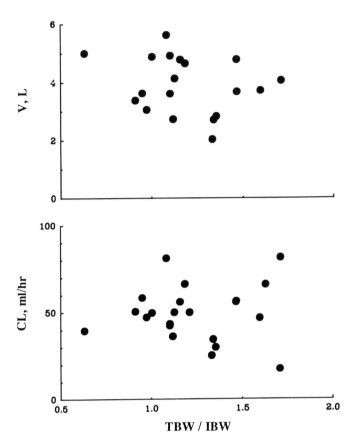

Figure 2 Relationships between volume of distribution (V) and clearance (CL) of ^{111}In-CYT-103 and the ratio of total:ideal body weights (TBW/IBW) in the study patients.

better curve fitting and lower values of AIC (Table 4). Since free ^{111}In is known to be cleared rapidly from plasma [12], the detected plasma radioactivity is assumed to be due to ^{111}In bound to antibody. This assumption was not tested in the present study, but previous work with ^{111}In-CYT-103 provides supporting data. For example, Harwood et al. used Sephadex G-100 size exclusion chromatography to show that this ^{111}In-labeled MAb remains predominantly intact in human serum up to 8 days postinfusion [11]. This is also consistent with earlier unpublished data. Therefore, the half-life of ^{111}In in plasma probably reflects the half-life of the intact radiolabeled antibody.

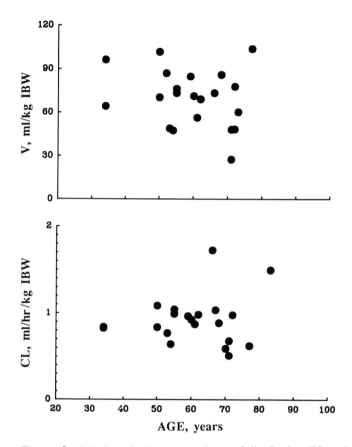

Figure 3 Relationships between volume of distribution (V) and clearance (CL) of ^{111}In-CYT-103 and age of the study patients.

The volume of distribution of ^{111}In-CYT-103 averaged 3.8 ± 1.2 liters and although small (about 7% of body weight), was larger than the plasma volume (4% of body weight). Studies of the distribution of immunoglobulins in rats [13,14] have shown that IgG is able to cross the membrane between the plasma and extravascular space. However, the large size of antibody molecules probably slows the rate of diffusion across such barriers, with the result that several days are required to attain a significant concentration in target sites. The distribution phase in some of the plasma data in this study may be related to the extravascular diffusion of the conjugate.

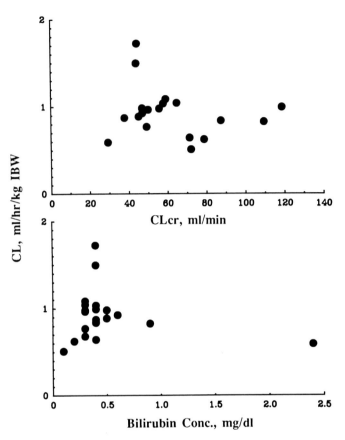

Figure 4 Relationships between clearance (CL) of ^{111}In-CYT-103 and creatinine clearances (CLcr) and serum bilirubin concentrations of the study patients.

^{111}In-CYT-103 conjugate intravenously administered to ovarian cancer patients was found to have a low systemic clearance averaging about 50 ml/hr, renal clearance averaging 4.9 ± 2.1 ml/hr, and a low fractional urinary elimination (about 10% of the systemic clearance). This low renal clearance is consistent with the suggestion that the major elimination pathway of IgG is via metabolism [15]. The organ or organs that account for this clearance are not known. Metabolism of antibodies by liver, spleen, lymph nodes, gut, kidney, and tumors has been reported [16]. Evidence of accumulation of MAb B72.3 in animal liver and spleen [4,12,17] and the fact that the primary metabolic site of gamma globulin in humans is liver [14] suggest that the liver, specifically hepatocytes

[18,19], may be the major metabolic site of elimination of ^{111}In-CYT-103. On the other hand, the limited variability in CL found in these patients could be explained by hypothesizing multiple sites of metabolism of ^{111}In-CYT-103. In the present study, neither hepatic function (as indicated by bilirubin level), renal function (CL_R), obesity, nor age affected the disposition of the antibody. However, this was a small, diverse group of subjects, and additional patients with extreme pathophysiology should be studied to properly assess the role organ dysfunctions might play in antibody metabolism.

REFERENCES

1. Nuti M, Teramoto YA, Mariani-Constantini R, et al. A monoclonal antibody (B72.3) defines patterns of distribution of a novel tumor-associated antigen in human mammary carcinoma cell populations. Int J Can 1982; 29:539–45.

2. Stramignoni D, Bowen R, Atkinson B, Schlom J. Differential reactivity of monoclonal antibodies with human colon adenocarcinomas and adenomas. Int J Cancer 1983; 31:543–52.

3. Thor A, Ohuchi N, Szpak CA, Johnston WW, Schlom J. Distribution of oncofetal antigen tumor-associated glycoprotein-72 defined by monoclonal antibody B72.3. Cancer Res 1986; 46:3118–24.

4. Yokoyama K, Carrasquillo JA, Chang AE, et al. Differences in biodistribution of indium-111- and iodine-131-labeled B72.3 monoclonal antibodies in patients with colorectal cancer. J Nucl Med 1989; 30:320–7.

5. Rodwell JD, Alvarez VL, Lee C, et al. Site-specific covalent modification of monoclonal antibodies: in-vitro and in vivo evaluations. Proc Natl Acad Sci USA 1986; 86:2632–6.

6. Metzler CM, Elfring, GK, McEwen AL. A package of computer programs for pharmacokinetic modeling in vivo. Biometrics 1974; 30:562–3.

7. Jusko WJ. Guidelines for collection and analysis of pharmacokinetic data. In: Evans WE, Schentag JJ, Jusko, WJ, eds. Applied pharmacokinetics. Spokane, WA:Applied Therapeutics, 1986:9–54.

8. Devine BJ. Gentamicin therapy. Drug Intell Clin Pharm 1974; 8:650–5.

9. Cockcroft DW, Gault MH. Prediction of creatinine clearance from serum creatinine. Nephron 1976; 16:31–41.

10. Akaike H. An information criterion. Math Sci 1976; 14:5–9.

11. Harwood SJ, Carroll RG, Webster WB, et al. Human biodistribution of ^{111}In-labeled B72.3 monoclonal antibody. Cancer Res 1990; 50:932s–936s.

12. Eger RR, Covell DG, Carrasquillo JA, et al. Kinetic model for the biodistribution of an ^{111}In-labeled monoclonal antibody in humans. Cancer Res 1981; 47:3328–36.

13. Dewey WC. Vascular-extravascular exchange of ^{131}I plasma proteins in the rat. Am J Physiol 1959; 197:423–31.

14. Waldman TA, Strober W. Metabolism of immunoglobulins. Progr Allergy 1969; 13:1–110.

15. Sands H, Jones PL. Methods for the study of the metabolism of radiolabeled monoclonal antibodies by liver and tumor. J Nucl Med 1987; 28:390–8.

16. Brown BA, Comeau RD, Jones PL, et al. Pharmacokinetics of monoclonal antibody B72.3 and its fragments labeled with either ^{125}I or ^{111}In. Cancer Res 1987; 47:1149–54.

17. Sands H, Jones PL. Methods for the study of the metabolism of radiolabeled monoclonal antibodies by liver and tumour. J Nucl Med 1987; 28:390–8.

18. Davidson BR, Boulos PB, Porter JB. Inhibition of the hepatocyte uptake of radiolabelled monoclonal antibodies by chelating agents. Eur J Nucl Med 1990; 17:294–8.

11

A Practical Approach to Planar and SPECT Imaging of ^{111}In-CYT-103

**B. David Collier, LisaAnn Trembath, Yu Liu,
H. Turgut Turoglu, Neetin Patel, and Shekhar Thakur**
Medical College of Wisconsin, Milwaukee, Wisconsin

INTRODUCTION

For the past 2 years, diagnostic studies using ^{111}In-CYT-103 have been performed at the Medical College of Wisconsin. Practical experience with both planar and SPECT imaging has been gained. Our initial experience with scintigraphic imaging of ^{111}In-CYT-103 was marked by technical problems to be overcome and pitfalls to be avoided. The physicians and technologists at the Medical College of Wisconsin would like to share the benefit from this 2-year experience with others. We hope that our current imaging protocols, which are designed to expedite patient imaging while avoiding, or at least minimizing, technical difficulties, will be of value to others.

The techniques described in this chapter are appropriate for use at both academic institutions and community hospitals. These protocols from the Medical College of Wisconsin can be implemented on the single detector rotating gamma cameras provided by most commercial vendors. We have attempted to provide a generic description of these techniques. However, some modifications may be in order before these protocols are put to routine use on the SPECT instrumentation at other institutions.

Only basic planar and SPECT techniques directed toward detection and localization of colorectal carcinoma are described in this chapter. Other worthwhile approaches, which use instrumentation not generally available to community hospitals, are not described. However, we anticipate that in the future, such significant advances as multidetector SPECT systems, more sophisticated subtraction and enhancement techniques, three-dimensional displays, and quantitation will be widely employed [1].

THE ROLE OF SPECT IMAGING

High-quality planar imaging of ^{111}In-CYT-103 often is sufficient (see Fig. 1). For example, in the patient scheduled for resection of hepatic metastates, ^{111}In-CYT-103 often is used to detect potential extrahepatic sites of disease, thereby changing the surgical approach. If planar imaging detects such extra-

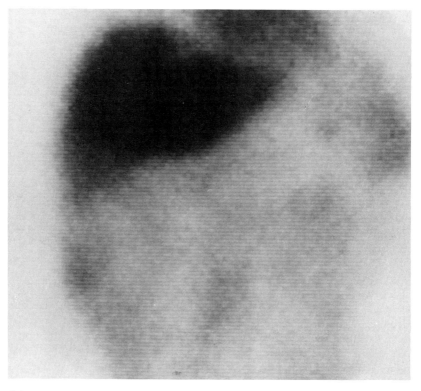

(a)

Figure 1 Sixty-year-old man with recurrent right upper quadrant and midabdominal carcinoma 2 years following abdominoperineal resection of a rectal carcinoma. Anterior planar images of the abdomen at 48 hr (a) and 96 hr (b) show substantial interval

hepatic sites of metastatic colorectal carcinoma, then it is not necessary to proceed on to SPECT. Although from a practical point of view all patients will not require SPECT imaging, the research protocols at the Medical College of Wisconsin have emphasized both SPECT and planar imaging for all ^{111}In-CYT-103 examinations. In our experience, SPECT contributes significantly to diagnostic efficacy in approximately one-third of cases. (Figs. 2–4).

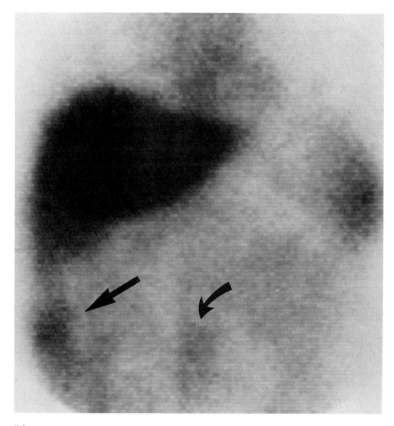

(b)

Figure 1 Continued

clearing of blood pool and gut activity. Sites of surgically confirmed carcinoma in the right side of the abdomen (straight arrow) and midabdomen (curved arrow) are more obvious on the 96-hr image. Preoperative computed tomography scan was normal.

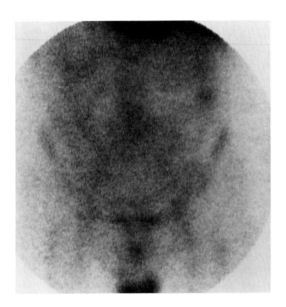

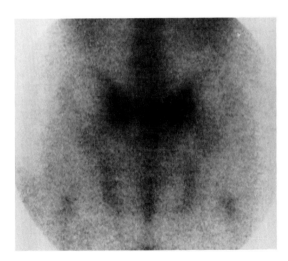

(b)

Figure 2 Sixty-eight-year old man with a 3-cm adenocarcinoma of the mid-ascending colon. 168-hr delayed anterior (a) and posterior (b) planar images show uptake by the lesion in part obscured by residual gut and background activity. Uptake at the

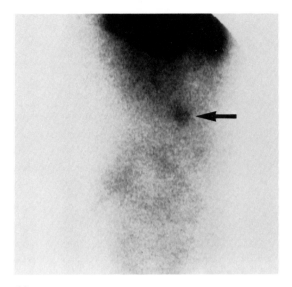

(c)

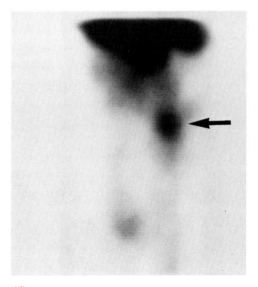

(d)

site of adenocarcinoma is better seen on right lateral planar view (c) (arrow). Sagittal SPECT image (d) through the right lobe of the liver and the ascending colon convincingly demonstrates abnormal uptake in the tumor (arrow).

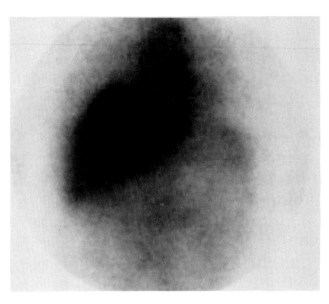

(a)

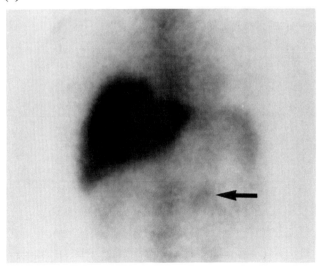

(b)

Figure 3 Fifty-eight-year-old woman with circumferential "apple core" adenocarcinoma of the transverse colon. Because of background activity, uptake by lesion is not evident on 72-hr anterior planar image (a) and is only faintly seen on 120-hr anterior planar

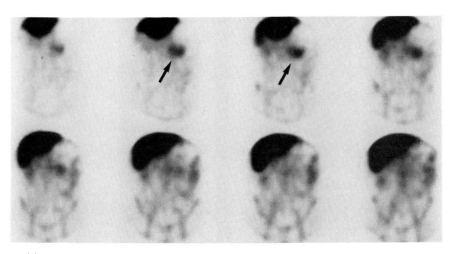

(c)

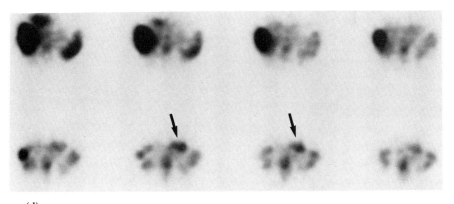

(d)

image (b) (arrow). Selected coronal (c), transaxial (d), and sagittal (e) SPECT images more clearly demonstrate intense uptake of ^{111}In-CYT-103 by the adenocarcinoma (arrows).

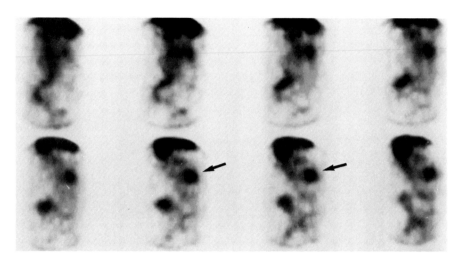

(e)

Figure 3 Continued

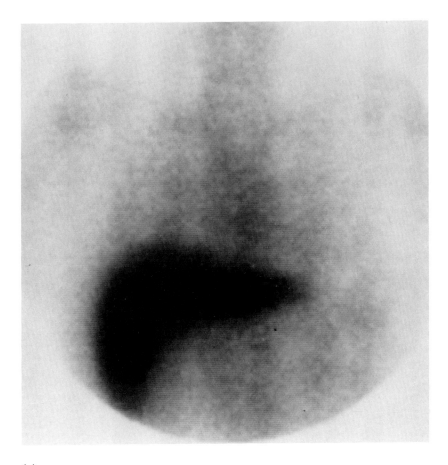

(a)

Figure 4 Forty-two-year-old man 1 year status post transverse colectomy and splenectomy for colon carcinoma. Computed tomography (CT) scan 1 year after surgery showed the new finding of a 3-cm metastasis centrally located in the right lobe of the liver. ^{111}In-labeled CYT-103 study was undertaken to identify any extrahepatic metastases in this patient who was a candidate for resection of the hepatic lesions. Anterior view planar image of chest and upper abdomen at 120 hr (a) in addition to all other planar views was normal. Sequential transaxial SPECT images through the liver and upper abdomen (b) show faint but definitely abnormal uptake in the left upper quadrant (arrows). CT did not identify left upper quadrant tumor, but extrahepatic metastatic disease at this site was confirmed at the time of laparotomy.

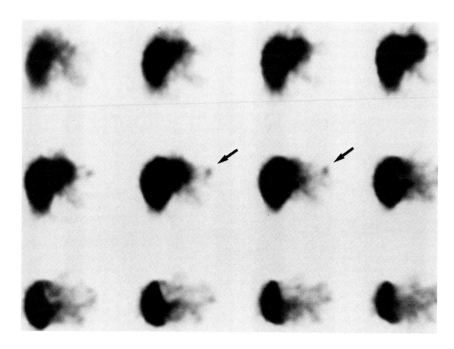

(b)

Figure 4 Continued

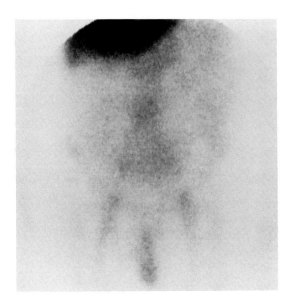

(a)

Figure 5 Eighty-eight-year-old man with 8-cm obstructing sigmoid carcinoma metastatic to liver and para-aortic lymph nodes. Planar images at 48 hr (a) and 144 hr (b) in addition to coronal SPECT images at 144 hr (c) show no uptake at the site of extrahepatic disease. Computed tomography also failed to demonstrate extrahepatic disease while showing liver metastases that were confirmed at surgery.

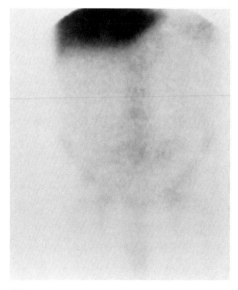

(b)

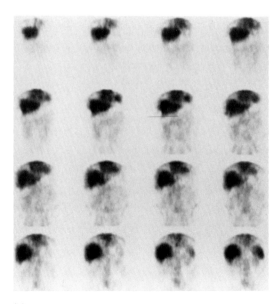

(c)

Figure 5 Continued

However, some patients with bulky extrahepatic disease will not be identified by either planar or SPECT ^{111}In-CYT-103 imaging (Fig. 5).

SPECT removes from the diagnostic image activity arising both in front and behind the tomographic plane of medical interest. For example, when used to detect uptake of ^{111}In-CYT-103 at extrahepatic sites of metastatic colorectal carcinoma, coronal SPECT images detect only the activity arising in the cross-sectional plane containing the lesion. Unwanted underlying activity arising in such structures as the spine, vessels, and kidneys, in addition to unwanted overlying activity in loops of bowel, is removed from the SPECT image. This removal of unwanted underlying and overlying activity both increases image contrast and provides additional three-dimensional positional information. It has been shown that SPECT is of value for detecting and localizing lesions [2–9].

TECHNIQUES FOR PLANAR AND SPECT IMAGING

A quality control program appropriate for planar and SPECT imaging of ^{111}In-CYT-103 is shown in Table 1. This quality control program is intended as a practical, easily executed safeguard against such problems as nonuniformity artifacts, inappropriate center-of-rotation artifacts, and poor-quality studies due to lack of spatial resolution. Methods for ^{111}In-CYT-103 kit preparation and quality control currently in use at the Medical College of Wisconsin are listed in Table 2. Once technologists become familiar with these procedures,

Table 1 Quality Control for Planar and SPECT Imaging of ^{111}In-CYT-103

Day of imaging:	Extrinsic flood with medium-energy collimator and [57]Co sheet source: 3.0 million counts for 400-mm FOV camera. 4.5 million counts for 500-mm FOV camera.
Weekly:	1. Intrinsic (no collimator) uniformity flood with ^{111}In point source: 3.0 million counts for 400-mm FOV camera. 4.5 million counts for 500-mm FOV camera. 2.30 million count extrinsic flood for uniformity correction using medium energy collimator and [57]Co sheet source.
Every other week:	Update center of rotation
Monthly:	1. Image bar phantom using ^{111}In point source. No collimator. Collect 2.0 million counts. 2. Image ^{111}In-filled tomographic phantom (optional).

Table 2 Kit Preparation and Quality Control

Kit preparation
1. One-half hour prior to the labeling procedure, take the CYT-103 kit out of the refrigerator and bring to room temperature.
2. Add 0.5 ml sodium acetate to the ^{111}In vial. Mix carefully.
3. Inject between 5 and 6 mCi of the buffered ^{111}In into the CYT-103 vial. Mix and incubate at room temperature for 30 min.
4. Filter the solution with a 0.22-μm filter by attaching the filter to a 10-ml syringe and drawing up the contents of the reaction vial.

Quality control
1. Materials: ITLC paper, 0.9% sodium chloride, and 0.05 molar DTPA.
2. Mix 75 μl of the ^{111}In-CYT-103 with 75 μl of 0.05 M DTPA. Allow to stand at room temperature for 1 min.
3. Fill a test tube with 0.9% sodium chloride solution to a depth of about 0.5 cm.
4. Spot a small drop of the DTPA-treated product onto an ITLC strip 1 cm from the bottom (origin).
5. Place the spotted strip in the solvent.
6. Allow the saline front to migrate 10 cm from the origin (approximately 2–4 min).
7. Remove the strip and cut in half. Count each half-strip in a gamma counter.
8. Radiochemical purity = [cpm in bottom/(cpm in bottom + cpm in top)] x 100.
9. To be acceptable for injection, radiochemical purity of the preparation must be greater than 90%.

preparation and quality control of ^{111}In-CYT-103 can be accomplished routinely in no more than 45 min.

Attention should also be diverted to patient preparation (Table 3) and the precautions needed to guard against potential allergic reactions (Table 4). Before beginning to infuse a patient with ^{111}In-CYT-103, physicians at our institution insist that a 1-mg dose of epinephrine for intravenous injection be prepared. This epinephrine might be necessary for the rapid treatment of an anaphylactic reaction. Fortunately, no life-threatening allergic reactions have occurred at the Medical College of Wisconsin or any other institutions participating in ^{111}In-CYT-103 protocols. Minor allergic reactions, such as fever, chills, itching, changes in blood pressure, sweating, and skin rashes, occur in less than 5% of patients.

Table 3 Patient Preparation, Precautions, and ^{111}In-CYT-103 Injection

1. Explain to the patient the potential allergic reactions and other risks of injecting a foreign protein.
2. Obtain a detailed history of allergies and previous exposure to murine antibodies.
3. Record baseline vital signs (temperature, pulse rate, respiratory rate, and blood pressure).
4. Have epinephrine available to treat anaphylaxis.
5. Have a crash cart within ready access and a physician available at the time of injection.
6. Slowly inject between 4.5 and 5.5 mCi of ^{111}In-CYT-103. The entire dose should be injected over 5 min. Use a heparinized saline flush to keep the i.v. line open.
7. Obtain vital signs at 5, 15, 30, and 60 min postinjection.

Table 4 Potential Adverse Reactions to ^{111}In-CYT-103

Most frequent adverse reactions
  1. Fever
  2. Chills
  3. Hypotension and hypertension
  4. Itching
  5. Rash
  6. Sweating

Infrequent adverse reactions
  1. Chest pain
  2. Difficulty focusing
  3. Dizziness
  4. Headache
  5. Nausea
  6. Flushing
  7. Hypothermia
  8. Angioedema
  9. Temporary joint pain and tenderness

Potential severe adverse reactions
  1. Anaphylaxis
  2. Serum sickness with fever, urticaria, lymphadenopathy, arthralgias, and renal dysfunction.

Standard protocols for planar and SPECT imaging of ^{111}In-CYT-103 are given in Tables 5 and 6. We have found that patient convenience and treatment schedules make it difficult to hold to a rigid schedule for imaging. In particular, we frequently obtain images more than 96 hr after injection. High background activity on 48-hr images often suggests that late delayed images will have enhanced diagnostic value [10,11]. When using a 500-mm camera, a single SPECT study can encompass likely sites of metastatic disease in the abdomen and pelvis. When using a 400-mm camera, two SPECT studies that together encompass the entire abdomen and pelvis may be necessary. In addition, if planar images raise the question of disease in the chest or other extra-abdominal site, additional SPECT should be obtained.

Table 5 Planar Imaging Protocol

Collimator:	Medium energy
Energy:	173 and 247 Kev; 20% window
Matrix:	256 x 256 (128 x 128 can be used)
Imaging sequence:	Acquire planar images at 48 and between 96 and 144 hr postinjection.
Images acquired:	Anterior chest, abdomen, and pelvis
	Posterior chest, abdomen, and pelvis
	Lateral views as may be requested
Time per image:	10 min

Hints
1. Empty colostomy or urine collection bag before scanning.
2. Mark colostomy sites with ^{111}In or lead markers.
3. Use same positioning for 48- and 96-hr images.
4. Position gamma camera as close to the body as possible.
5. Acquire detailed patient history, especially noting previous surgeries.
6. Be consistent in positioning and try to image all patients in the same way.

Table 6 SPECT Imaging Protocol

Acquisition Protocol

Imaging sequence:	Acquire SPECT between 96 and 144 hr postinjection.
Energy:	173 and 247 Kev; 20% window
Collimator:	Medium energy
Orbit:	360°, elliptical stepwise; 64 views
Matrix:	128 x 128 (64 x 64 can be used on a 400-mm FOV camera)
Time per view:	40 sec

Reconstruction protocol
1. Uniformity correction.
2. Hanning filter (frequency cutoff = 0.5 cycle/cm) before backprojection.
3. Tomographic reconstruction by filtered backprojection with ramp filter and no attenuation correction. Create 3-pixel-thick transaxial tomograms.
4. Create 3-pixel-thick sagittal and coronal tomograms.
5. Display tomographic images using a linear gray scale.

Hints
1. If patient is agitated or in pain, acquire SPECT study for only 30 sec per view.
2. When displaying and filming SPECT of pelvis, lower the upper threshold enough to see vascular structures.

Common technical problems encountered by physicians and technologists at the Medical College of Wisconsin are listed in Table 7. Particularly notable are the need for meticulous patient positioning, markers to identify colostomy and urine bag sites, maneuvers to deal with background and colon activity, and concern for patient comfort.

Before beginning SPECT imaging of ^{111}In-CYT-103, our institution had an experience with over 5000 SPECT studies. However, we initially found SPECT imaging of monoclonal antibodies to be extremely challenging. Optimal quality control, methods that guard against the most serious pitfalls, and appropriate protocols for data acquisitions and processing have since been introduced. At this time, we feel that ^{111}In-CYT-103 planar and SPECT imaging can routinely be performed as a high-volume procedure at both academic institutions and community hospitals.

Table 7 Common Technical Problems

Problem	Solution
Colon activity	To identify colon activity, compare 48- and 96-hr images; bowel prep can be given between first and second imaging times
Activity at colostomy site or urine collection bag site	Mark site on planar images with ^{111}In or lead marker; acquire lateral images; collection bags should be emptied before each imaging session
[57]Co-point source marker does not show up on images	Use ^{111}In point source or lead marker
Positive neck nodes	Include neck on anterior chest view; image patient with no pillow, neck in slight extension, and head completely straight; head tilt could obscure uptake in lymph nodes
High liver activity	Inherent to ^{111}In antibody imaging; acquire chest image with only tip of liver in view; acquire pelvis image with only bottom edge of liver in view; this prevents chest and pelvis images from being saturated with counts from liver
High renal activity	Delayed imaging reduces amount of blood pool activity in the kidneys
High body background	Delayed imaging required; best times usually are between 48 and 96 hr; however, delayed images out to 144 hr may be obtained
Bone marrow activity	Seen with most ^{111}In-labeled antibodies; useful for identifying bony anatomy
Long imaging times	Make patient as comfortable as possible; use pillows under knees to relieve strain on lower back; as necessary, support the arms with straps and arm boards; allow patient to sit up or walk around between planar and SPECT imaging
Few anatomical landmarks, leading to difficulty in	Position exactly the same for 48- and 96-hr images; to produce bilaterally symmetrical

Table 7 Continued

interpreting the study	positioning, tie the feet together for views of the pelvis; be consistent and image every patient the same way
Poor-quality SPECT images	Patient motion is the most frequent cause for poor-quality SPECT; ask patients to lie very still on the table; explain importance of remaining motionless
^{111}In-CYT-103 uptake at sites of surgical anastomoses	Obtain detailed patient history with particular emphasis on previous surgeries
Intravascular activity that does not clear over time	Slow clearance of ^{111}In-CYT-103 from the vascular space may be responsible

REFERENCES

1. Logan KW. Quantitative SPECT imaging for diagnosis and dosimetry in radionuclide therapy. Int J Rad Appl Instrum (B) 1987; 14(3):205–9.
2. Berche C, Mach J-P, Lumbroso J-D, Langlais C, Aubrey F, Bucheggar F, Carrel S, Rougier P, Parmentier C, Tubiana M. Tomoscintigraphy for detecting gastrointestinal and medullary thyroid cancers: first clinical results using radiolabelled monoclonal antibodies against carcinoembryonic antigen. Br Med J 1982; 285:1447–51.
3. Epenetos AA, Britton KE, Mather S, Shepherd J, Granowska M, Taylor-Papadimitriou J, Nimmon CC, Durbin H, Hawkins LR, Malpas JS, Bodmer WF. Targeting of iodine-123-labelled tumour associated monoclonal antibodies to ovarian, breast and gastrointestinal tumours. Lancet 1982; 2:999–1004.
4. Montz R, Klapdor R, Kremer B, Rothe B. Immunoscintigraphy and SPECT in patients with pancreatic cancer. Nuklearmedizin 1985; 24(5–6):232–7.
5. Bischof-Delaloye A, Delaloye B, Buchegger F, von Fliedner V, Mach JP. Immunoscintigraphy of CEA producing tumors with special emphasis on the use of MAB fragments and ECT. In: Nuclear medicine in clinical oncology: current status and future aspects. 1986:150–5.
6. Abdel-Nabi HH, Schwartz AN, Goldfogel G, Ortman-Nabi JA, Matsouka DM, Under MW, Wechter DG. Colorectal tumors: scintigraphy with In-111 anti-CEA monoclonal antibody and correlation with surgical, histopathologic, and immunohistochemical findings. Radiology 1988; 166(3);747–52.
7. Patt YZ, Lamki LM, Haynie TP, Unger MW, Rosenblum MG, Shirkboda A, Murray JL. Improved tumor localization with increasing dose of Indium-111 labeled anti-carcinoembryonic antigen monoclonal antibody ZCE-025 in metastatic colorectal cancer. J Clin Oncol 1988; 6(8):1220–30.

8. Kramer EL, Sanger JJ, Walsh C, Kanamuller H, Unger MW, Halverson C. Contributions of SPECT to imaging of gastrointestinal adenocarcinoma with In-111 labeled anti-CEA monoclonal antibody. Am J Radiol 1988; 151(4):697–703.

9. Perkins AC, Whalley DR, Ballantyne KC, Pimm MV. Gamma camera emission tomography using radiolabelled antibodies. Eur J Nucl Med 1988; 14:45–9.

10. Carrasquillo JA, Sugarbaker P, Colcher D, Reynolds JC, Esteban J, Bryant G, Keenan AM, Perentesis P, Yokoyama K, Simpson DE, Ferroni P, Farkas R, Schlom J, Larson SM. Radioimmunoscintigraphy of colon cancer with iodine-131-labelled B72.3 monoclonal antibody. J Nucl Med 1988; 29:1022–30.

11. Halpern SE, Haindl W, Beauregard J, Hagan P, Clutter M, Amox D, Merchant B, Under N, Mongovi C, Bartholomew R, Jue R, Carlo D, Dillman R. Scintigraphy with In-111 labelled monoclonal antitumor antibodies: kinetics, biodistribution, and tumor detection. Radiology 1988; 168:529–36.

12

Future Directions in Tumor Radioimmuno-detection

Thomas J. McKearn
CYTOGEN Corporation, Princeton, New Jersey

INTRODUCTION

Monoclonal antibodies directed toward tumor-associated antigens and radiolabeled with gamma-emitting radionuclides can make a significant contribution to the diagnosis and clinical management of human malignancies. The B72.3-containing immunoscintigraphic agents described in this volume provide an excellent illustration of the clinical utility of radiolabeled monoclonal antibodies in the management of colorectal and ovarian carcinomas. Although not presented here, encouraging preliminary findings suggest that monoclonal antibodies, labeled with therapeutic radionuclides, can also be useful for cancer treatment [1–3].

Despite the successful application of monoclonal antibody technology for tumor radioimmunodetection, limitations associated with existing immunoscintigraphic agents suggest that further research efforts in this field are warranted. As shown in Table 1, many of the problems with currently available monoclonal antibody–based imaging agents involve low target-to-nontarget localization ratios which limit the sensitivity of these agents, especially for small (<1 cm) tumor deposits and tumors that express small amounts of the target antigen [1,4–6]. In addition, the immunogenicity associated with the administration of nonhuman proteins may reduce the utility of subsequent

Table 1 Radiolabeled Monoclonal Antibodies (MAbs) for Tumor Detection: Current Problems, and Potential Solutions

Problems with existing MAb-base imaging agents	Potential areas for improvement					
	MAb	labeling method/linker	Radiolabel	Tumor characteristics	Host characteristics	Imaging technology
Inadequate MAb delivery to tumor site	x	x		x	x	x
High background radiolocalization	x	x	x	x	x	x
Tumor antigenic heterogeneity	x			x		
MAb immunogenicity	x				x	
Low sensitive for small (<1 cm) tumor lesions	x	x	x	x		x

doses of these agents [7,8] and may interfere with the tumor marker assays used for monitoring a patient's response to antitumor therapy [9,10].

Strategies involving modification of the radiolabeled immunoconjugates, manipulation of tumor and/or host characteristics, and advances in imaging technologies (Table 1) are being pursued to overcome these problems. These research efforts are directed toward the optimization of safe and effective immunoscintigraphic agents that can accurately define the location and extent of primary and metastatic disease, including lesions missed by existing diagnostic modalities, and that can be repeatedly administered to monitor for disease recurrence and response to therapy. These research strategies will be reviewed in an attempt to predict the future of tumor radioimmunodetection.

STRATEGIES FOR IMPROVING TUMOR RADIOIMMUNODETECTION
Targeting Agents: Antibodies and Antibody-like Molecules

Many early clinical investigations in tumor radioimmunodetection utilized whole antibodies as the targeting components of immunoscintigraphic agents. Although encouraging clinical results have been obtained using whole antibody-based imaging agents, concern about the development of human antimouse antibodies (HAMA) associated with these agents and their less than optimal pharmacokinetic characteristics has fostered research efforts aimed at developing other types of targeting molecules [11,12].

Making Monoclonal Antibodies More Human

The strategy for overcoming the immunogenicity of monoclonal antibody preparations has focused on developing human or human-like antibody molecules for radioimmunodetection. The results of these investigations include chimeric, humanized, and human antibodies.

A chimeric antibody results from a fusion of the genes responsible for encoding the variable regions of murine antibodies with genes encoding the structure of human antibody constant regions [13]. The interspecies murine/human chimeric antibodies expressed using this technology retain the antigen-binding specificity of the murine monoclonal antibody. Since the constant region domains of the chimera consist of the human peptide sequences, these hybrid antibodies were predicted to be less immunogenic than the parent murine immunoglobulins. Evidence in support of this contention has been obtained in clinical studies involving administration of a chimera of monoclonal antibody 17-1A, which demonstrated a positive anti-idiotype response in only 1 in 10 patients; this comares with an immune response of 70%, including 25% having an anti-idiotype response, in patients treated with murine 17-1A monoclonal antibody [14]. However, similar constructs prepared using the V_H and V_L pairs from the monoclonal antibody B72.3 have elicited a high proportion of HAMA responses [15]. Hence, it is not currently possible to predict which chimeric antibodies will show decreased HAMA responses.

Another approach used to produce antibody constructs that are even more human-like involves transplantation of murine hypervariable regions, the complementarity determining regions (CDRs) that comprise the antigen-binding sites, into human immunoglobulin genes [16]. Again, the immunogenic potential of the resulting "humanized" antibodies, which contain human constant and variable region frameworks and murine CDRs, is predicted to be low. Additionally, with this approach there is a greater possibility of failing to confer the desired affinity to the "humanized" antibody, presumably as a consequence of the contribution of variable region frameworks to the topography of the engrafted CDRs. Daily doses of CAMPATH-1H, a humanized IgG1, have been administered to two patients for the treatment of lymphoma. The preliminary findings showed evidence of remission in both patients; neither patient exhibited detectable antimouse antibodies [17]. However, since these patients were probably immunocomprised as a result of their disease and since the CAMPATH-1H antibody itself may be immunosuppressive, further investigation of the immunogenic potential of this and other similar agents is needed.

The logical extension of these strategies for humanizing murine antibodies is the production of human monoclonal antibodies. In addition to having a lower immunogenic potential, human antibodies may recognize epitopes that are not detected by non-human antibodies, and, therefore, have different or expanded specificities compared to their murine counterparts [18,19]. Although technological limitations of in vitro immunization methods previously led to difficulties in the production of these agents, recent developments in these techniques have made human monoclonal antibody production a viable strategy [18]. Alternatively, transgenic expression systems may be used to produce human monoclonal antibodies [20].

Whereas chimeric, humanized, and human monoclonal antibodies may provide solutions to the problem of HAMA, these constructs may have pharmacokinetic characteristics, including increased blood half-lives, that are less optimal for external imaging applications than whole murine immunoglobulins [14,21]. These longer-acting antibodies with lower immunogenic potential may, therefore, be most useful as immunotherapeutic agents.

Creating Smaller Antibody-Based Targeting Agents

The large size (approximately 150,000 daltons for IgG) of intact immunoglobulins results in slow clearance from the blood pool and slow and limited diffusion into tumor tissues. As a consequence of this biodistribution profile, imaging

MOLECULAR ENGINEERING OF RECOGNITION SYSTEMS

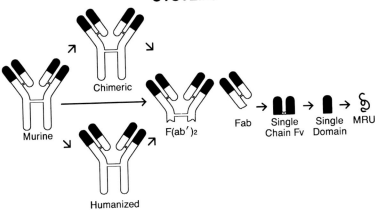

Figure 1 Strategies for altering the targeting vehicle of monoclonal antibody–based imaging agents include the development of chimeric and humanized monoclonal antibodies and the use of antibody fragments and even smaller immunoreactive molecules. (Reprinted with permission from Ref. 11.)

with intact antibodies must be delayed, often for several days after administration, until the circulating radiolabeled antibody is cleared from the blood pool. Moreover, the tumor-to-background radiolocalization ratios tend to be less than optimal for the visualization of smaller tumor lesions [5,12]. One approach to these problems is the production of smaller antibody-based targeting components that retain the specificity of whole antibodies but clear more rapidly from the blood and penetrate target tissues more readily. As shown in Figure 1, such constructs include antibody fragments, single-chain antibodies, and even smaller peptides [11]. Obviously, these antibody-based targeting agents can be produced from antibody chimeras and humanized antibodies as well as murine immunoglobulins.

Various antigen-binding fragments can be produced through enzymatic digestion of monoclonal antibodies (Fig. 1). Papain removal of the Fc or constant region of IgG antibodies yields two Fab fragments, each of which contains an antigen-combining region, whereas pepsin digestion removes part of the Fc region and produces a F(ab')$_2$ fragment, containing two antigen-binding sites. Removal of the Fc portion of the immunoglobulin also has the advantage of making fragments less immunogenic than intact antibodies. In certain situations, these smaller immunoreactive molecules may be preferable for radioimmunodetection, since blood pool clearance is more rapid, resulting in the earlier achievement of higher target-to-background ratios, which in turn permits earlier imaging times [22–24].

Extending this approach to even smaller antibody-based targeting components has resulted in Fv fragments, which are pairs of specific variable light- and heavy-chain regions produced using protein engineering techniques [25,26]. Other investigators have connected the light- and heavy-chain variable regions using a peptide linkage to form single-chain antibodies with antigen-binding characterisitcs similar to those of the parent whole antibody [27–29]. In an effort to achieve the simplest possible immunoreactive species, the peptide sequences of single CDRs have been evaluated [30,31]. Preliminary results with CDRs indicate that some of these small peptides mimic the antigenic specificity of the whole antibodies from which they were derived. The study of these CDRs may faciliate the preparation of small molecular recognition units (MRUs) consisting of low-molecular-weight immunoreactive peptides using protein engineering techniques [11]. Indeed, the utility of MRUs for radioimmunodetection has been demonstrated in preclinical models of thrombus imaging, suggesting these new constructs may increase our knowledge of antigen-antibody interactions and perhaps lead to further innovations in targeted delivery of cancer diagnostic and therapeutic agents.

Other Approaches for Increasing Tumor Targeting

The strategies described above offer the potential for increasing the tumor targeting of monoclonal antibodies and antibody-based constructs used for radioimmunodetection. However, targeting tumor deposits that either do not express the target antigen or contain only small amounts of the antigen remains problematic [32,33], even for immunoscintigraphic agents with improved pharmacokinetic characteristics. A potential solution to this problem is the development of antibodies directed against antigen targets that are contained in higher concentrations and/or are unique to tumor cells. One such agent exploits the high degree of necrosis that characterizes cancer tissues and targets the histones of dying or necrotic cells [34]; this approach may prove particularly useful for radioimmunotherapy of large solid tumors. Alternatively, administration of a "cocktail" of antibodies, each directed against a different tumor-associated antigen, may increase the number of antibody-binding sites within a given tumor and thereby improve immunoscintigraphic sensitivity [35,36]. An extension of this approach is the preparation of patient-specific cocktails based on the antigenic determinants of individual tumors [1]. Finally, regional administration of monoclonal antibodies [37] to increase the concentration at the tumor site (e.g., i.p. administration for tumors confined to the peritoneal cavity) or administration of clearing antibody (HAMA) to reduce the background concentration of the first antibody [38] has been successfully employed to improve the tumor-to-background ratio for radioimmunodection.

Selection of Radionuclides for Immunoscintigraphy

Several radionuclides have been used for labeling monoclonal antibodies for tumor radioimmunodetection (Table 2). There is no ideal gamma-emitting isotope for immunoscintigraphy. Rather, the choice of radionuclide is dependent several factors, including the photon energy of the radionuclide and the compatibility of its half-life of radioactive decay and the pharmacokinetic profile of the monoclonal antibody targeting vehicle. Additional considerations involve the relative cost and availability of potentially useful radionuclides, as well as the availability of effective labeling methodologies [1,39]. Using the most appropriate radionuclide for the targeting vehicle is another mechanism for optimizing image quality and improving the accuracy of radioimmunodetection.

The iodine isotopes ^{131}I and ^{123}I have been used extensively for radioimmunodection. The well-established chemistries of these isotopes permit effective labeling to monoclonal antibodies for imaging. The long half-life of ^{131}I is well suited to its use with intact monoclonal antibodies, which require longer equilibration times prior to imaging in order to achieve optimal tumor-to-background ratios. However, the ß-emission energy of ^{131}I limits the imaging dose of this isotope. The gamma energy of ^{123}I is more favorable for radioimmunodetection, and its short half-life is compatible with the pharmacokinetic profile of antibody fragments. However, since ^{123}I must be obtained from a reactor, its short half-life becomes an economic disadvantage. The in vivo metabolism of the iodine isotopes results in dehalogenation, an additional disadvantage of these radioisotopes [39,40].

For whole antibody-based imaging agents, the chemistry techniques used to produce stable ^{111}In chelates and the favorable gamma energies of ^{111}In help to overcome some of the problems associated with radioiodinated agents. In spite of the extensive uptake of this radionuclide by the reticuloendothelial system and its relatively higher cost, ^{111}In may be the radionuclide of choice for intact monoclonal antibody imaging agents [12,39,41]. However, the extensive liver and spleen uptake of ^{111}In-labeled antibodies reduces their ability to detect tumors in these organs.

^{99m}Tc is the most favored radionuclide for many applications of external gamma camera imaging. Its low cost and ready availability, its favorable gamma emission energy, and its short half-life make ^{99m}Tc an excellent choice for use with monoclonal antibody fragments and even smaller antibody-based constructs [12,39]. The disadvantages of ^{99m}Tc-labeled agents include extensive kidney uptake, which may obscure tumor depostis in the abdomen, and its relatively short half-life, which limits the acquisition of follow-up images at time points

Table 2 Characteristics of Isotopes Used for Radioimmunodetection

Isotope	Gamma emission energy (Kev)	Radioactive half-life	Advantages	Disadvantages
^{99m}Tc	141	6 hr	Decay energy Availability Cost	Labeling chemistry Kidney uptake Limited follow-up imaging
^{123}I	159	13 hr	Decay energy Labeling chemistry	Availability Cost In vivo dehalogenation Decreased immunoreactivity
^{111}In	171 245	68 hr	Decay energy Chelation chemistry	Cost Uptake in RES
^{131}I	364	8 days	Labeling chemistry Availability	Decay energy In vivo dehalogenation Decreased immunoreactivity

later than 18–24 hr postinfusion. In the future, the increased use of smaller antibody-like molecules for external scintigraphy as well as the refinement of chemical radiolabeling methods and improved gamma camera imaging technology, both of which will be discussed in subsequent sections of this chapter, may lead to the expanded use of ^{99m}Tc for tumor radioimmunodetection.

Methods for Radiolabeling Antibodies for Immunoscintigraphy

The method used to link the monoclonal antibody and the radionuclide is an important determinant of the absolute amount of radioactivity delivered to the tumor and, therefore, the tumor-to-background ratio. A variety of techniques have been used for in vitro radiolabeling of monoclonal antibodies and antibody fragments [39,42]. Moreover, strategies for in vivo radiolabeling are currently being investigated [42–45]. As with the choice of radionuclides for imaging, there is no single labeling method that is ideal for all monoclonal antibody–based immunoscintigraphic agents. The selection of appropriate labeling methods depends on the radionuclide and its in vivo disposition, as well as the antibody or antibody-based targeting vehicle and the availability of its functional groups for providing a point of attachment or derivitization [39]. Methods of choice are "user friendly," so that they can be performed successfully and reproducibly by radiopharmacy and nuclear medicine personnel; result in linkages that are stable in vivo; and do not reduce the immunoreacitivity of the targeting vehicle.

As shown in Table 3, in vitro approaches for linking radioisotopes and monoclonal antibodies can be divided into direct labeling and labeling with chelating agents. In general, radioiodination of antibodies is accomplished through direct labeling, whereas metallic radionuclides, which have limited affinity for the antibody-targeting vehicles, are linked to antibodies through

Table 3 Methods for Labeling Monoclonal Antibodies for Radioimmunodetection

Labeling approach	Isotope(s)
Direct labeling	^{131}I, ^{123}I, ^{99m}Tc
Labeling with chelating agents	^{111}In, ^{99m}Tc
Random conjugation	
Site-specific conjugation	
In vivo labeling	^{111}In
Antichelate antibody	
Antibody avidin-biotin complexes	

bifunctional chelating agents [39,42]. Although ^{99m}Tc can be attached to antibodies using both methods, chelation techniques generally result in radiolabeled antibodies with greater in vivo stability. To date, the newer in vivo labeling methods, which utilize chelation chemistry, have only been used to produce ^{111}In-labeled immunoconjugates.

Direct Labeling Methods

Labeling antibodies with iodine isotopes involves oxidation of the iodine to the positively charged iodinium ion, which is then attached to the antibody via electrophilic substitution at the aromatic ring of tyrosine or histidine residues. The oxidizing agents most frequently employed for labeling monoclonal antibodies with ^{131}I or ^{123}I are lactoperoxidase, chloramine-T, and iodogen [42]. Although there are advantages and disadvantages of each of these methods, the iodogen method appears to give the highest radiolabeling yields and generally results in the most immunoreactive iodinated antibodies. All three labeling procedures are associated with some loss of immunoreactivity and, as noted previously, the resulting radioiodinated antibodies are subject to dehalogenation in vivo.

^{99m}Tc-labeled antibodies produced by some direct labeling methods also demonstrate in vivo instability. However, stable ^{99m}Tc-labeled antibodies can be produced using recently developed direct labeling techniques, including the Schwarz method [46]. In this approach, the antibody is reduced, lyophilized, and then reacted with ^{99m}Tc under reducing conditions.

Radiolabeling with Chelating Agents

Labeling monoclonal antibodies with radiometals is a two-stage process: conjugation of a bifunctional chelating agent to the antibody molecule followed by addition of the metallic radionulcide. Chelating agents used in the formation of radiolabeled immunoconjugates contain a functional group that forms a covalent linkage with the amino acid residues or oxidized carbohydrate moieties of the monoclonal antibody and a chelating group that binds the radiometal [39]. Ethylenediaminetetraacetic acid (EDTA), diethylenetriaminepentaacetic acid (DTPA), and derivatives of these chelators have been used to label monoclonal antibodies with radiometals; DTPA and DTPA derivatives are generally preferred because they form more stable chelates with metallic radionuclides. These reagents utilize the polyaminocarboxylic acid regions to complex the radiometal and various functional groups– includng a carboxylic anhydride, a diazonium ion, a bromoacetyl group, or other reactive group–to conjugate the antibody [42]. Because of the variety of functional groups, several different reactions have been used to covalently bind these chelators with the targeting agents.

In vivo stability of radiolabeled antibody conjugates is critical to effective tumor radioimmunodetection. Serum transferrin and other plasma proteins can remove radiometals from chelates [42]. Nonspecific uptake of the transchelated radiometals by the liver or other organs can reduce the diagnostic utility of monoclonal antibody immunoconjugates for tumors located in or near these organs. In an effort to bind radiometals tightly under physiological conditions, derivatives of polyazamacrocycles have been employed as chelating agents [47,48]. Preliminary results indicate that macrocyclic chelates are less sensitive to acid-catalyzed dissociation and, therefore, more inert in the liver and the stomach, which have a lower pH [48]. The initial clinical imaging results with macrocyclic chelates of monoclonal antibodies are also encouraging [47].

Most of the conjugation methods described above permit random attachment of the chelator to various amino acid residues, including those located in the antigen-binding region of the monoclonal antibody molecule. Such methods can change the affinity of the targeting vehicle for the tumor antigen, thereby reducing the immunoreactivity of the resulting antibody conjugate [39]. To overcome this problem, site-specific conjugation methods for antibodies [49] and antibody fragments [50] have been developed. The method of Rodwell et al. [49] is based on the finding that carbohydrate moieties are generally located exclusively on the Fc portion of the antibody molecule, distal to the antigen-binding region. Using covalent chemistry techniques, these investigators conjugated the antibody and a linker-chelator at the oxidized oligosaccharide moieties. Unlike random conjugation methods, this site-specific approach produces monoclonal antibody conjugates that retain the homogeneous antigen-binding characteristics and affinity of the native antibody, and that demonstrate more efficient in vivo tumor targeting [49]. To conserve the immunoreactivity of Fab' fragments, which are often less reactive than F(ab')$_2$ fragments, site-specific conjugation of the sulfhydryl group of Fab' fragments has been accomplished by Ishikawa et al. [50] using a maleimide function.

In Vivo Radiolabeling Methods

Although tumor targeting with antibodies occurs quite rapidly, high background radioactivity generally prevents the early visualization of tumor deposits. Thus, delays of several days, during which the radiolabeled antibody is cleared from the blood pool, are needed to optimize the tumor-to-background ratios. In an effort to increase the absolute amount of the radiolabel delivered to the tumor and the blood pool clearance of circulating radiolabel, strategies for in vivo labeling of monoclonal antibodies have been devised [43–45].

One approach to in vivo labeling involves the initial administration of unlabeled monoclonal antibodies or antibody fragments with dual specificities, that is, one combining site directed against the tumor antigen and the other against a low-molecular-weight chelate of the gamma-emitting radionuclide [43]. After a time delay, during which tumor targeting and blood pool clearance have proceeded to achieve a high tumor-to-background ratio, the radiolabeled chelate is injected. External scintigraphy can then be performed soon after injection of the labeled chelate [51]. An alternative method involves the administration of unlabeled monoclonal antibody conjugated with biotin, followed by radiolabeled avidin or streptavidin or an initial injection of avidin-conjugated antibody followed by administration of radiolabeled biotin [44]. Studies in tumor-bearing animals have confirmed the feasibility of this approach [44,45].

Tumor and Host Characteristics: Implications for Radioimmunodetection

Modifications of the antibody-targeting vehicle, the radiolabel, and the chemical linkage between these two components have been explored to improve the sensitivity and specificity of tumor radioimmunodetection. An alternative strategy is modulation of selected tumor and/or host characteristics that influence the tumor delivery and uptake of radiolabeled monoclonal antibodies. The results of animal and clinical studies have identified several of these variables, including tumor size, tumor vascularization and vascular permeability, and amount of the specific antigen expressed by the tumor [52–56]. Strategies for modulating many of these variable are being investigated by several groups (Table 4); some of these approaches have shown promise for improving tumor radioimmunodetection with monoclonal antibodies.

As the delivery system for radiolabeled monoclonal antibodies, the tumor vasculature is a major determinant of tumor uptake of immunoscintigraphic agents. Studies in animal models have demonstrated a direct correlation between tumor blood flow and xenograft uptake of radiolabeled antibodies. These experiments also showed that vascular permeability can limit the tumor uptake of immunoscintigraphic agents, with the rate of vessel transit being inversely related to the size of the targeting molecule [53,57]. Strategies for manipulating these determinants of antibody uptake are complicated by the finding that tumor blood flow tends to be lower and tumor vasculature less uniform than that of normal tissues [57]. This is especially true for larger tumors with necrotic centers. As a result, on a per-weight basis, smaller tumors accumulate larger amounts of radiolabeled antibodies than larger tumors [54].

To date, efforts aimed at improving delivery of radiolabeled monoclonal antibodies to tumors by increasing tumor blood flow and vascular permeability

Table 4 Modulations of Tumor and/or Host Characteristics to Improve Tumor Uptake of Radiolabeled Monoclonal Antibodies (MAbs)

Factors that limit MAb uptake by tumors	Strategies for manipulating limiting factors to increase tumor uptake of MAbs

Limited tumor vasculature
Blood flow
Vascular permeability
	Hyperthermia
	External-beam radiation
	Pharmacological agents
	  Alpha-adrenergic agonists
	  Beta-adrenergic antagonists
	  ACE inhibitors + angiotensin II
	  Osmotic agents (mannitol)
	  Biological response modifiers
	  Interleukins
	  Tumor necrosis factor

Large tumor size	External-beam radiation Cytoreductive treatment Surgery Chemotherapeutic agents
Limited tumor antigen expression	Interferons

have met with only minimal success. Treatment of athymic mice using either hyperthermia or external-beam radiation has produced modest increases in tumor localization of monoclonal antibodies [58]. Subsequent studies have indicated that the enhanced tumor uptake associated with external-beam radiation did not result from an independent effect on tumor blood flow or vascular permeability, but rather was related to the reduction in tumor mass produced by irradiation [52]. Although these findings are not particularly encouraging for radioimmunodetection, they may have important implications for cancer radioimmunotherapy using monoclonal antibodies. These data suggest that the optimal setting for using antibodies labeled with therapeutic radioisotopes may be as adjuvant therapy in patients with small tumor deposits or those at high risk of local or distant tumor recurrence. In patients with bulky disease, radiolabeled monoclonal antibodies could be utilized after surgical, radiation, or chemotherapeutic treatments have been employed to reduce tumor mass.

As shown in Table 4, various pharmacological agents have been administered to increase the tumor uptake of radiolabeled monoclonal antibodies by increasing tumor blood flow and/or vascular permeability [59,60]. Both alpha-adrenergic agonists and beta-adrenergic antagonists have been administered to tumor-bearing animals in an attempt to increase the tumor-to-blood ratio of radiolabeled monoclonal antibodies. Only the latter treatment resulted in augmentation of the localization ratio, and the increase was due to a reduction in the amount of radiolabeled antibody in the blood rather than increased uptake by the tumor [59]. Administration of mannitol to patients with metastatic melanoma resulted in modest increases in delivery of a radiolabeled antibody fragment into the central nervous system [60]. Yamaguchi et al. [61] reported that administration of enalapril, a potent kininase inhibitor, in combination with angiotensin II resulted in increased delivery of monoclonal antibody A7 to colon cancer xenografts in nude mice. In spite of the rather modest improvements in tumor delivery using pharmacological agents in combination with monoclonal antibodies, further investigation of this approach appears warranted. One potentially promising strategy involves coadministration of radiolabeled monoclonal antibodies and biological response modifiers that have vasoactive properties, including interleukins and tumor necrosis factor.

Central to these attempts at perfecting a regimen for altering the vascular permeability in nude mouse xenografts is the assumption that these rapidly growing xenograft tumors have vascular beds that resemble physiologically and/or pharmacologically the vascular compartments of autochthonous tumors in patients. The development of a preclinical tumor model with a vascular compartment which mimics that found in patients would represent an important contribution to this field.

Another strategy for increasing tumor uptake of monoclonal antibodies involves augmentation of tumor antigen expression. Data from human cancer cell lines and from biopsies of in situ cancer lesions indicate that tumor antigens often may be expressed by only a fraction of the tumor cells in any particular lesion [55]. Thus, heterogeneous expression of tumor antigens can limit specific tumor localization of monoclonal antibody–based imaging agents. In vitro studies, experiments with human tumor xenografts in animal models, and human clinical trials have demonstrated that administration of recombinant human interferons, specifically alpha- and gamma-interferons, can up-regulate the expression of some human tumor antigens, including CEA and TAG-72, thereby improving tumor localization by radiolabeled monoclonal antibodies [56,62,63]. Because the interferons are potent immunomodulators and demonstrate a multiplicity of biological effects, these preliminary results are particularly encouraging since the enhanced antigenic expression was elicited using low doses of these agents. Coadministration of interferons appears to be a promising approach for improving the sensitivity of radioimmunodetection using monoclonal antibodies. If further experimentation confirms the success of this approach for improving tumor targeting, it may be especially relevant for radioimmuno-therapy using monoclonal antibodies.

Although the strategies discussed for the modulation of tumor or host characteristics offer promise for improving antibody-directed targeting, further investigation is needed to assess the magnitude of improvement associated with each approach versus the risk of coadministration of other pharmaceutical, radiopharmaceutical, or biological agents. Moreover, as our knowledge of tumor immunology and physiology increases, it is likely that a number of new options will emerge for improving the tumor uptake of radiolabeled antibodies.

Advances in Immunoscintigraphic Technology and Equipment

Optimizing tumor-to-background localization ratios through improvements in the immunoscintigraphic agents themselves or through modulation of tumor or host determinants of tumor uptake will undoubtedly increase the clinical utility of radioimmunodetection using monoclonal antibodies. The effective application of state-of-the-art nuclear medicine technology to tumor radioimmunodetection using monoclonal antibodies is another strategy for improving the diagnostic accuracy of these agents [64,65].

New developments in nuclear medicine include improved software for processing of digital imaging data and hardware for the acquisition of high-resolution planar and single photon emission tomographic (SPECT) antibody images [64–66]. Other technological advances that can be applied to tumor radioimmunodetection with monoclonal antibodies include positron emission tomgraphic (PET) scanning [6,67], creation of fusion images from SPECT images and computerized tomographic (CT) or magnetic resonance imaging (MRI) scans [68,69], and the intraoperative use of gamma-detecting probes [70,71].

The quality of gamma camera images can be improved by applying various data-processing techniques. Optimal image processing can improve the sensitivity and specificity of immunoscintigraphy by enhancing image contrast and resolution. Standard data-processing techniques include filtering, i.e., a smoothing process to reduce statistical fluctuations that can hinder image analysis; choice of the color or gray display scale and selection of upper and lower limits of the scale; and image subtraction, a technique for reducing nonspecific radiolocalization [64]. Effective utilization of any or all of these technqiues can make images easier to analyze by increasing the tumor-to-background radiolocalization, thereby enhancing the tumor detection rate as well as the specificity of antibody imaging. For example, compared with the conventional or default approach, an algorithm tailored specifically to ^{111}In-labeled antibody images and designed to set the upper and lower limits of the color scale used for image display resulted in a significant improvement in imaging sensitivity [72].

Incorrect or inappropriate utilization of data-processing methods can result in uninterpretable images. As nuclear medicine physicians gain experience with monoclonal antibody–based imaging agents and become familiar with the various patterns of normal tissue and nonspecific uptake associated with the radioisotopes and targeting vehicles, their ability to process and interpret these images will improve. Moreover, as radiolabeled monoclonal antibody-based imaging agents improve, the importance of optimal image-processing techniques will diminish. At present, however, appropriate processing of digital imaging data is one way of improving the quality of the diagnostic information obtained from immunoscintigraphic agents.

When used in conjunction with standard planar scintigraphy, SPECT imaging generally results in higher tumor detection rates, especially for smaller tumor lesions, for monoclonal antibody–based imaging agents, and more accurate anatomical localization of tumor lesions detected on the planar images [73,74]. Further, SPECT imaging facilitates comparison of the result of antibody images and CT scans. Technological developments in SPECT imaging, including multiple-detector systems linked to graphics supercomputers, should further increase the utility of SPECT for tumor radioimmunodetection [66]. The new multihead SPECT systems demonstrate improved resolution as well as shorter image acquisition times; the latter feature substantially reduces the time that sick patients must lie still in uncomfortable, and often painful, positions to complete a SPECT study and dramatically increases the throughput of a nuclear medicine service. The use of supercomputers for processing the digital data from these SPECT units allows three-dimensional reformatting, high-resolution graphical displays, and faster and simultaneous data acqusition and image reconstruction [66]. Application of this new SPECT technology will improve the quality and, therefore, enhance the utility of antibody images.

Correlation between the results of antibody imaging, which produces high-contrast, functional scans as a result of specific tumor antigen binding, and the precise anatomical scans resulting from MRI or CT imaging has been facilitated by image fusion, the computer-assisted combination of the two images [68,69]. Compared with the manual comparison of antibody and CT scans, image fusion allows more precise anatomical-functional correlation and facilitates the quantitation of areas of interest [75]. When used to compare monoclonal antibody scans and CT images, this technique enabled the identification of the anatomical site of radiolabeled antibody uptake, permitted the easy identification of nonspecific radiolocalization in normal tisuses and structures, and helped to accurately characterize equivocal findings on the individual studies [69].

Another technological innovation that has been utilized for tumor with radioimmunodetection with monoclonal antibodies is the hand-held gamma-detecting probe [71,71]. This device has been successfully used during surgery to examine areas suspicious for tumor and facilitate biopsy and/or resection of sites of radiolocalization. Through the use of intraoperative probes, the sensitivity of external scintigraphy may be enhanced with respect to small tumor deposits located deep in the body. Moreover, using the probe to examine the margins of surgical resection may enable more complete surgical dissection of tumor lesions. Finally, use of the gamma-detecting probe during the pathological examination of resected tissue may facilitate tissue sectioning, thereby improving the accuracy of histopathological staging.

At present, most clinical trials with monoclonal antibodies for tumor radioimmunodetection utilize gamma scintigraphy; however, the use of PET scanning is being investigated for antibody imaging [6,67]. Although the high cost and small number of PET cyclotron facilities has limited the clinical use of this technology, PET scanning can calculate absolute tissue levels of radiolabel, information that cannot be obtained from gamma scintigraphy, and this information may be utilized to make accurate dosimetric estimates for radioimmunotherapy. In an animal model system, the utility of PET scanning has been demonstrated for tumor detection using monoclonal antibodies radiolabeled with a positron-emitting isotope [67]. If ongoing clinical studies confirm these findings and if the problems of high cost and limited availability can be overcome, PET scanning may increase the amount and value of the diagnostic information generated from monoclonal antibody–based imaging agents.

CONCLUSION

The value of immunoscintigraphy using radiolabeled monoclonal antibodies has already been demonstrated for the selective recognition of tumor lesions. The problems associated with the currently available agents–suboptimal tumor-to-background ratios, HAMA development, antigenic heterogeneity, etc.–are gradually being overcome through appropriate research efforts. This chapter outlines some of the approaches directed toward improving the quality and enhancing the utility of monoclonal antibody immunoscintigraphy. By exploring several different strategies to improve tumor radioimmunodetection using monoclonal antibodies, we are not only increasing the probability of success, but also accelerating the development of the related fields of molecular biology, recombinant technology, nuclear medicine, and tumor immunology. The pace of research and development in these fields is so rapid that a comprehensive description of the future of tumor radioimmunodetection is not only impossible, but is likely to be obsolete at the time of its publication.

The diagnosis and staging of cancer using radiolabeled monoclonal antibodies has advanced from the research laboratory to the clinical management of cancer patients. It seems fair to expect that within the decade of the 1990s, the enormous potential of monoclonal antibodies will begin to be realized.

REFERENCES

1. Keenan AM. Radiolabeled monoclonal antibodies: current status and future outlook. In: Nuclear Medicine Annual. New York: Raven Press, 1988:171–207.
2. Kuzel TM, Zimmer AM, Duda RB, et al. Phase I trial of intravenously administered Y-90 labeled B72.3 monoclonal antibody in patients with refractory B72.3 reactive adenocarcinomas. Antibody Immunoconjugates Radiopharmaceu 1990; 3:53.
3. Order SE, Sleeper AM, Stillwagon GB, et al. Current status of radioimmunoglobulins in the treatment of human malignancy. Oncology 1989; 3:115–20.
4. Sands H. Radioimmunoconjugates: an overview of problems and promises. Antibody Immunoconjugates Radiopharmaceut 1988; 1:213–26.
5. Bradwell AR, Fairweather DS, Dykes PW, Keeling A, Vaughn A, Taylor J. Limiting factors in the localization of tumours with radiolabelled antibodies. Immunol Today 1985; 6:163–70.
6. McAfee JG, Kopecky RT, Frymoyer PA. Nuclear medicine comes of age: its present and future roles in diagnosis. Radiology 1990; 174:609–20.
7. Perkins AC, Pimm MV, Powell MC. The implications of patient antibody response for the clinical usefulness of immunoscintigraphy. Nucl Med Commun 1988; 9:273–82.
8. Reynolds JC, Del Vecchio S, Sakahara H, et al. Antimurine antibody response to mouse monoclonal antibodies: clinical findings and implications. Nucl Med Biol 1989; 16:121–5.
9. Muto MG, Lepisto EM, VandenAbbeele AD, Knapp RC, Kassis AI. Influence of human antimurine antibody on CA 125 levels in patients with ovarian cancer undergoing radioimmunotherapy or immunoscintigraphy with murine monoclonal antibody OC 125. Am J Obstet Gynecol 1989; 161:1206–12.
10. Morton BA, O'Connor-Tressel M, Beatty BG, Shively JE, Beatty JD. Artifactual CEA elevation due to human anti-mouse antibodies. Arch Surg 1988; 123:1242–6.
11. Rodwell JD. Engineering monoclonal antibodies: a perspective of the future. Nature 1989; 342:99–100.
12. Larson SM, Carrasquillo JA, Reynolds JC. Radioimmunodetection and radioimmunotherapy. Cancer Invest 1984; 2:363–81.
13. Morrison SL, Johnson MJ, Herzenberg LA, Oi VT. Chimeric human antibody molecules: mouse antigen-binding domains with human constant region domains. Proc Natl Acad Sci USA 1984; 81:6851–5.

14. LoBuglio AF, Wheeler RH, Trang J, et al. Mouse/human chimeric monoclonal antibody in man: Kinetics and immune response. Proc Natl Acad Sci USA 1989; 86:4220–4.

15. Meredith R, Orr R, Grizzle W, et al. Comparative localization of murine and chimeric B72.3 antibody in patients with colon cancer. Antibody Immunoconjugates Radiopharmaceut 1991; 4:207.

16. Jones PT, Dear PH, Foote J, Neuberger MS, Winter G. Replacing the complementarity-determining regions in a human antibody with those from a mouse. Nature 1986; 321:522–5.

17. Hale G, Clark MR, Marcus R, et al. Remission induction in non-Hodgkin lymphoma with reshaped human monoclonal antibody CAMPATH-1H. Lancet 1988; 2:1394–9.

18. Borreback CAK. Human mAbs produced by primary in-vitro immunization. Immunol Today 988; 9:355–9.

19. Schlom J, Wunderlich D, Teramoto YA. Generation of monoclonal antibodies reactive with human mammary carcinoma cells. Proc Natl Acad Sci USA 1980; 77:6841–5.

20. Richa J, Lo CW. Introduction of human DNA into mouse eggs by injection of dissected chromosome fragments. Science 1989; 245:175–7.

21. Morrison SL. Transfectomas provide novel chimeric antibodies. Science 1985; 229:1202–7.

22. Carrasquillo JA, Krohn KA, Beaumier P, et al. Diagnosis of and therapy for solid tumors with radiolabeled antibodies and immune fragments. Cancer Treat Rep 1984; 68:317–28.

23. Buraggi GL, Callegaro L, Mariani G, et al. Imaging with ^{131}I-labeled monoclonal antibodies to a high-molecular-weight melanoma-associated antigen in patients with melanoma: efficacy of whole immuoglobulin and its F(ab')$_2$ fragments. Cancer Res 1985; 45:3378–87.

24. Buchegger F, Haskell CM, Schreyer M, et al. Radiolabeled fragments of monoclonal antibodies against carcinoembryonic antigen for localization of human colon carcinoma grafted into nude mice. J Exp Med 1983; 158:413–27.

25. Reichmann L, Foote J, Winter G. Expression of antibody Fv fragment in myeloma cells. J Mol Biol 1988; 203:825–8.

26. Skerra A, Pluckthun A. Assembly of a functional immunoglobulin Fv fragment in Escherichia coli. Science 1988; 240:1038–41.

27. Bird RB, Hardman KD, Jacobsen JW, et al. Single-chain antigen-binding proteins. Science 1988; 242:423–6.

28. Huston JS, Levinson D, Mudgett-Hunter M, et al. Protein engineering of antibody binding sites: recovery of specific activity in an anti-digoxin single-chain Fv analogue produced in Escherichia coli. Proc Natl Acad Sci USA 1988; 85:5879–83.

29. Ward ES, Gussaw D, Griffitha AD, Jones PT, Winter G. Binding activities of a repertoire of single immunoglobulin variable domains secreted from *Escherichia coli*. Nature 1989; 341:544–6.

30. Taub R, Gould RJ, Garsky VM, et al. A monoclonal antibody against the platelet fibrinogen receptor contains a sequence that mimics a receptor recognition domain in fibrinogen. J Biol Chem 1989; 264:259–65.
31. Williams WV, Moss DA, Kieber-Emmons T, et al. Development of biologically active peptides based on antibody structure. Pro Natl Acad Sci USA 1989; 86:5537–41.
32. Natali PG, Cavalieri R, Bigotti A, et al. Antigenic heterogeneity of surgically removed primary and autologous metastatic human melanoma lesions. J Immunol 1983; 131:508–13.
33. Horan Hand P, Nuti M, Colcher D, Schlom J. Definition of antigenic heterogeneity and modulation among human mammary carcinoma populations using monoclonal antibodies to tumor-associated antigens. Cancer Res 1983; 43:728–35.
34. Epstein AC, Chen FE, Taylor CR. A novel method for detection of necrotic lesions in human cancers. Cancer Res 1988; 48:5842–8.
35. Tagliabue E, Porro G, Barbanti P, et al. Improvement of tumor cell detection using a pool of monoclonal antibodies. Hybridoma 1986; 5:107–15.
36. Chatal JF, Saccavini JC, Fumoleau P, et al. Immunoscintigraphy of colon carcinoma. J Nucl Med 1984; 25:307–14.
37. Colcher D, Esteban J, Carrasquillo JA, et al. Complementation of intracavitary and intravenous administration of monoclonal antibody (B72.3) in patients with carcinoma. Cancer Res 1987; 47:4218–24.
38. Goodwin D, Meares C, Diamanti C, et al. Use of specific antibody for rapid clearance of circulating blood background from radiolabeled tumor imaging proteins. Eur J Nucl Med 1984; 9:209–15.
39. Bhargava KK, Seetharama AA. Labeling of monoclonal antibodies with radionuclides. Semin Nucl Med 1989; 19:187–201.
40. Order SE, Klein JL, Leichner PK, et al. Monoclonal antibodies: potential role in radiation therapy and oncology. Int J Radiat Oncol Biol Phys 1982; 8:1193–1201.
41. Anderson WT, Strand M. Radiolabeled antibody: iodine versus radiometal chelates: NCI Monogr 1987; 3:149–51.
42. Saccavini J, Bohy J, Bruneau J. Radiolabeling of monoclonal antibodies. In: Chatel JF, ed. Monoclonal antibodies in immunoscintigraphy. Boca Raton, FL:CRC Press, 1989:61–73.
43. Reardon DT, Meares CF, Goodwin DA, et al. Antibodies against metal chelates. Nature 1985; 316:265–8.
44. Hnatowich DJ, Virzi F, Rusckhowski M. Investigations of avidin and biotin for imaging applications. J Nucl Med 1987; 28:1294–1302.
45. Paganelli G, Pervez S, Siccardi AG, et al. Intraperitoneal radio-localization of tumors pre-targeted by biotinylated monoclonal antibodies. Int J Cancer 1990; 45:1184–9.
46. Schwarz A, Steinstrasser A. A novel approach to Tc-99m labeled monoclonal antibodies. J Nucl Med 1987; 28:721.
47. Meares CF, Moi MK, Diril H, et al. Macrocyclic chelates of radiometals for diagnosis and therapy. Br J Cancer 1990; 62:21–6.

48. Parker D. Tumour targeting with radiolabelled macrocycle-antibody conjugates. Chem Soc Rev 1990; 19:217–91.

49. Rodwell JD, Alvarez VL, Lee C, et al. Site-specific covalent modification of monoclonal antibodies: in vitro and in vivo evaluations. Proc Natl Acad Sci USA 1986; 83:2632–6.

50. Ishikawa E, Imagawa M, Haschida S, Yoshitake S, Hamaguchi Y, Uneo T. Enzyme labeling of antibodies and their fragments for enzyme immunoassay and immunohistochemical staining. J Immunoass 1983; 4:209.

51. Frincke JM, Chang CH, Ahlem CN, et al. Pharmacokinetics of bifunctional antibody delivered In-111 benzyl EDTA to colon tumors in nude mice. J Nucl Med 1986; 27:1042.

52. Wong JYC, Williams LE, Hill LR, et al. The effects of tumor mass, tumor age, and external beam radiation on tumor-specific antibody uptake. Int J Radiat Oncol Biol Phys 1989; 16:715–20.

53. Sands H, Jones PL, Shah SA, Palme D, Vessella RL, Gallagher BM. Correlation of vascular permeability and blood flow with monoclonal antibody uptake by human Clouser and renal cell xenografts. Cancer Res 1988; 48:188–93.

54. Hagan PL, Halpern SE, Dillman RO, et al. Tumor size: effect on monoclonal antibody uptake in tumor models. J Nucl Med 1986; 27:422–27.

55. Schlom J, Horan Hand P, Greiner JW, et al. Innovations that influence the pharmacology of monoclonal antibody guided tumor targeting. Cancer Res 1990; 50:820s–827s.

56. Grenier JW, Horan Hand P, Colcher D, et al. Modulation of human tumor antigen expression. J Lab Clin Med 1987; 109:244–61.

57. Sands H, Jones PL. Physiology of monoclonal antibody accretion by tumors. In: Goldenberg DM, ed. Cancer imaging with radiolabeled antibodies. Kluwer, 1990:97–122.

58. Stickney DR, Gridley DS, Kirk GA, Slater JM. Enhancement of monoclonal antibody binding with a single dose of radiation or hyperthermia. Cancer Drug Deliv 1985; 2:225.

59. McKenzie IFC, Smyth MJ, Kanellos J, Sacks NPM, Thompson CH, Pietersz GA. Preclinical studies with a variety of immunoconjugates. Presented at the Second International Conference on Monoclonal Antibody Immunoconjugates for Cancer, San Diego, CA, 1987.

60. Neuwelt EA, Sprecht HD, Barnett RA, et al. Increased delivery of tumor specific monoclonal antibodies to brain after osmotic blood-brain barrier modification in patients with melanoma metastatic to central nervous system. Neurosurgery 1987; 20:885–95.

61. Yamaguchi T, Takahashi T, Noguchi A, et al. Enhancement of antibody delivery to the human colon cancer transplanted in nude mice by the kininase inhibitor enalapril and angiotensin II. Antibody Immunoconjugates Radiopharmaceut 1990; 3:81.

62. Greiner JW, Guadagni F, Noguchi P, Pestka S, Colcher D, Fisher PB, Schlom J. Recombinant interferon enhances monoclonal antibody targeting of carcinoma lesions in vivo. Science 1987; 235:895–8.

63. Rosenblum MG, Lamki LM, Murray JL, Carlo DJ, Gutterman JU. Interferon-induced changes in pharmacokinetics and tumor uptake of ^{111}In-labeled antimelanoma antibody 96.5 in melanoma patients. J Natl Cancer Inst 1989; 80:160–5.

64. Liehn J-C. Data processing in immunoscintigraphy. In: Chatal J-F, ed. Monoclonal antibodies in immunoscintigraphy. Boca Raton, FL:CRC Press, 1989:75–100.

65. Garty II, Serafini AN, Sfakianakis GN. Radioimmunoscintigraphy may detect early cancer. Diagn Imaging 1989; 2:84–93.

66. Devous MD. Graphics supercomputer powers multiple detector SPECT unit. Diagn Imaging 1989; 6:152–5.

67. Snook DE, Rowlinson-Busza G, Sharma HL, Epenetos AA. Preparation and in vivo study of [124]I-labelled monoclonal antibody H17E2 in a human tumour xenograft model. A prelude to positron emission tomography (PET). Br J Cancer 1990; 62:89–91.

68. Kaplan IL, Swayne LC. Composite SPECT-CT images: technique and potential application in chest and abdominal imaging. Am J Roentgenol 1989; 52:865–6.

69. Kramer EL, Noz ME, Sanger JJ, Megibow AJ, Maguire GQ. CT-SPECT fusion to correlate radiolabeled monoclonal antibody uptake with abdominal CT findings. Radiology 1989; 172:861–5.

70. Sickle-Santanello BJ, O'Dwyer PJ, Mojzisik C, et al. Radioimmunoguided surgery using the monoclonal antibody B72.3 in colorectal tumors. Dis Colon Rectum 1987; 30:761–4.

71. Jager W, Feistel H, Paterok EM, Ronay G, Tulusan AH, Wolf F, Lang N. Resection guided by antibodies: a diagnostic procedure during second-look operation in ovarian cancer patients. Br J Cancer 1990; 62:18–20.

72. Liehn J-C, Hannequin P, Nasca S, Lebrun D, Fernandez-Valoni A, Valeyre J. Immunoscintigraphy with indium-111 labeled monoclonal antibodies: the importance of a good display method. Clin Nucl Med 1989; 14:187–91.

73. Kramer EL, Sanger JJ, Walsh C, Kanamuller MW, Halverson C. Contribution of SPECT to imaging of gastrointestinal adenocarcinoma with ^{111}In-labeled anti-CEA monoclonal antibody. Am J Roentgenol 1988; 151:697–703.

74. Perkins AC, Whalley DR, Ballantyne KC, Pimm MV. Gamma camera emission tomography using radiolabelled antibodies. Eur J Nucl Med 1988; 14:45–9.

75. Swayne LC, Kaplan IL. Image fusion in medicine: an overview using the CT–SPECT model. J Nucl Med Technol 1989; 17:31–5.

Index

Barium enema in presurgical staging of colorectal cancer, 90-91

Carcinoembryonic antigen (CEA), 1
  in pre-surgical staging of colorectal cancer, 91-92
Chelate-conjugated B72.3 IgG, preclinical analysis of, 36-38
Chelating agents, radiolabeling with, 220-221
Colonoscopy in presurgical staging of colorectal cancer, 90
Colorectal cancer:
  clinicopathological staging, 94-95
  imaging in surgical management of, 89-109
  imaging with ^{131}B72.3 MAb, 45-55
    antigen and antibody, 46
    imaging results, 47
    pharmacokinetics, 47-49
    study design, 46
    tissue correlation, 49-53

[Colorectal cancer]
  toxicity, 53
  MAb imaging of primary colorectal cancer, 95-99
  MAb imaging of recurrent/metastatic colorectal cancer, 99-105
  presurgical staging, 90-94
  MAb B72.3 immunoscintigraphy in follow-up of patients with, 57-71
  evaluation of labeled B72.3 immunoreactivity, 59
  imaging techniques, 60
  monoclonal antibody and labeling procedure, 58-59
  patient profile, 59
  radioimmunoscintigraphy protocol, 59
  tissue studies, 60-61
  OncoScint in patients with, 73-88
  ^{111}In-CYT-103 imaging: factors affecting imaging performance, 79-84
  ^{111}In-CYT-103 imaging: patient selection, 74-77
  ^{111}In-CYT-103 imaging: performance, 77-79

[Colorectal carcinoma]
safety and HAMA response, 84
summary, 84-85
Computed tomography (CT):
comparison of ^{111}In-CYT-103 imaging performance with, 83-84, 117-118
^{111}In-CYT-103 immunoscintigraphy in identification of ovarian cancer versus, 117-118
CT/MRI in presurgical staging of colorectal cancer, 93-94

Diethylenetriaminepentaacetic acid (DTPA), 9-10, 220
Dukes' classification in clinicopathological staging of colorectal cancer, 94-95

Ethylenediaminetetraacetic acid (EDTA), 220

Glycyltyrosyl-(N-E-diethylenetriamine-pentaacetic acid)-lysine (GYK-DTPA), 73

Human antimouse antibodies (HAMA), 16-17, 75
in patients receiving OncoScint, 84

Immunoglobulins
IgG, 3-4
IgM, 3
Imaging in the surgical management of colorectal cancer patients, 89-109
clinicopathological staging of colorectal cancer, 94-95
Dukes' staging, 94-95
tumor characteristics, 94

[Imaging in the surgical management of colorectal cancer patients]
MAb imaging of primary colorectal cancer, 95-99
MAb imaging of recurrent/metastic colorectal cancer, 99-105
abdominal and pelvic recurrence, 100-101
distant metastasis: lung, bone, 102-104
hepatic metastasis, 101
occult disease, 104-105
patient management, 105
surveillance strategy, 99-100
presurgical staging of colorectal cancer, 90-94
barium enema, 90-91
CEA, 91-92
colonoscopy, 90
CT/MRI, 93-94
ultrasound, 92-93
Immune system, origin of, 2-3
Immunopharmacokinetics of ovarian cancer patients, 177-189
discussion, 186-188
methods, 178-180
antibody administration, 178
assays, 178
patients, 178
pharmacokinetic analysis, 178-180
sampling procedures, 178
results, 181-185
patient data, 181
pharmacokinetics, 181-185
Immunoscintigraphy, history of, 6-7
^{111}In, 9-11
imaging with, 11-12
^{111}In-CYT-103 immunoscintigraphy in colorectal carcinoma patients, 74-84
design and statistical considerations, 74
factors affecting imaging performance, 79-84
comparison of ^{111}In-CYT-103 imaging with CT, 83-84
contribution of SPECT to antibody imaging performance, 80-83
effect of prior antitumor therapy on imaging performance, 80
serum levels of TAG-72 antigen, 80
tumor expression of TAG-72 antigen, 80
patient selection, 74-77
baseline evaluation, 75

[Immunoscintigraphy, history of]
demographic characteristics, 75
^{111}In-CYT-103 administration, 75
^{111}In-CYT-103 scan interpretation, 76-77
^{111}In-CYT-103 scintigraphy, 76
performance, 77-79
liver metastasis, 79
occult disease, 78-79
radinuclid selection, 7-12
sensitivity, specificity, and accuracy, 77-78
Iodinated B72.3 IgG:
preclinical analysis of, 32-33
radioimmunotherapy using, 33-36
Iodine isotopes, radionuclide
alternatives to, 7-12
alternatives: ^{111}In and ^{99m}Tc, 9-11
imaging with ^{111}In and ^{99m}Tc, 11-12
mass effects, 12
problems with iodine, 7-9

Liver metastases, ^{111}In-CYT-103 immunoscintigraphic detection of, 79

Magnetic resonance imaging (MRI) in presurgical staging of colorectal cancer, 93-94
Molecular engineering of recognition systems, 215
Monoclonal antibodies (MAb), 23
imaging of primary colorectal cancer, 95-99
imaging of recurrent/metastatic colorectal cancer, 99-105
abdominal and pelvic recurrence, 100-101
distant metastasis: lung, bone, 102-104
hepatic metastasis, 101
occult disease, 104-105
patient management, 105
surveillance strategy, 99-100
intact as fragment, 12-14
production of, 4-6
Monoclonal antibody in colorectal carcinoma patients, 73-88
^{111}In-CYT-103 imaging:

factors affecting imaging performance, 79-84
patient selection, 74-77
performance, 77-79
safety and HAMA response, 84
summary, 84-85
Monoclonal antibody B72.3 (MAb B72.3), 23-44
analysis of recombinant/chimeric forms of B72.3, 39-41
augmentation of tumor antigen expression, 26-27
characterization of the TAG-72 antigen, 27-29
discussion, 68-69
distribution of TAG-72 expression 24-25
immunoscintigraphy in colorectal cancer patient follow-up, 57-71
evaluation of labeled B72.3 immunoreactivity, 59
imaging techniques, 60
monoclonal antibody and labeling procedure, 58-59
patient profile, 59
radioimmunoscintigraphy protocol, 59
tissue studies, 60-61
preclinical analysis of chelate-conjugated B72.3 IgG, 36-38
radioimmunoscintigraphic studies of patients with colon cancer, 61-67
radioimmunotherapy using iodinated B72.3 IgG, 33-36
serum assays for TAG-72, 29-32
TAG-72 expression in cell lines versus tumors, 25-26
MAb ^{131}B72.3, imaging of colorectal carcinoma with, 45-55
antigen and antibody, 46
imaging results, 47
pharmacokinetics of, 47-49
study design, 46
tissue correlation, 49-53
toxicity, 53

Occult disease:
detection by ^{111}In-CYT-103
immunoscintigraphy, 78-79, 118-120

[Occult disease]
   MAb imaging of recurrent/metastatic
      colorectal cancer and, 104-105
OncoScint image atlas in patients with
      colorectal or ovarian malignancies,
      141-175
   areas of inflammation, 172-174
   breast nipple shadows, 175
   carcinomatosis, 153
   colostomy sites, 169
   isolated pelvic recurrences, 150-152
   metachronous recurrence, 152
   nonspecific bowel patterns, 168
   normal OncoScint distribution, 142-143
   ovarian carcinoma-patterns of recurrence,
      162-165
   ovarian fibroma, 166-167
   patterns of bony metastases, 154-156
   patterns of hepatic metastases, 148-149
   patterns of recurrence-brain metastases,
      157
   patterns of recurrence-miscellaneous, 159
   primary colorectal cancer, 144-147
   primary ovarian cancers, 160-161
   urinary bladder, 171
Ovarian cancer, 111-124
   diagnosis and staging of, 125-140
   immunopharmacokinetics of, 177-189
      discussion, 186-188
      methods, 178-180
      results, 181-185
   materials and methods, 112-114
      efficacy and safety analyses, 114
      patient population, 112
      preparation of ^{111}In-CYT-103, 113-114
      study plan, 112-113
   results, 114-121
      detection of occult disease by ^{111}In-CYT-
         103 immunoscintigraphy, 118-120
      ^{111}In-CYT-103 imaging sensitivity and
         specificity, 114-117
      ^{111}In-CYT-103 immunoscintigraphy versus
         CT, 117-118
      patient characteristics, 114
      safety of ^{111}In-CYT-103 infusion, 120-121
   surgical management of, 125-140
      antibody imaging: potential impact on
         patient management (results), 132
      antibody imaging performance versus
         patient management impact (results),
         132-136
      diagnosis and staging, 125-126

[Ovarian cancer]
   discussion and results, 137-138
   ^{111}In-CYT-103   immunoscintigraphy,
      127-128
   methods, 128-130
   patient population, surgical findings,
      and antibody imaging results, 130-132
   requirements for new nonsurgical diagnos-
      tic approaches for ovarian cancer,
      126-127

Planar imaging, 191-192
   techniques for, 192-209
      imaging protocol, 206
      kit preparation and quality control, 204
      patient preparation and precautions,
         205
      potential adverse reactions to
         ^{111}In-CYT-103, 205
      quality control of planar imaging of
         ^{111}In-CYT-103, 204
      technical problems, 207-208

Radioimmunoimaging, 1-22
   future directions, 16-18
   history of immunoscintigraphy, 6-7
   IgG molecule, 3-4
   intact antibody versus fragments for RID,
      12-14
   origin of the immune system, 2-3
   production of a monoclonal antibody, 4-6
   radionuclide alternatives to isotopes of
      iodine, 7-12
      alternatives: ^{111}In and ^{99m}Tc, 9-11
      imaging with ^{111}In and ^{99m}Tc, 11-12
      mass effects, 12
      problems with iodine, 7-9
   relevance of basic tumor and normal tissue
      physiology to successful RID, 14-16
Radiolabeling antibodies for immunoscinti-
      graphy, 219-222
   direct labeling methods, 220
   in vivo radiolabeling methods, 221-222
   radiolabeling with chelating agents,
      220-221

Radionuclides for immunoscintigraphy, selection of, 217-219
Recombinant chimeric forms of B72.3, analysis of, 39-41
Recurrent/metastatic colorectal cancer, MAb imaging of, 99-105

SPECT imaging, 191-192
contribution to antibody imaging performance, 80-83
role of, 192
techniques for, 192-209
imaging protocol, 206
kit preparation and quality control, 204
patient preparation and precautions, 205
potential adverse reactions to ^{111}In-CYT-103, 205
quality control of SPECT imaging of ^{111}In-CYT-103, 204
technical problems, 207-208

[99m]Tc, 9-11
imaging with, 11-12
TAG-72 antigen, 24-25
characterization of, 27-29

[TAG-72 antigen]
enhancement of expression, 26-27
expression in cell lines versus tumors, 25-26
serum assays for, 29-32
Tissue physiology relevance to successful radioimmunodetection, 14-16
Tumor-associated antigens (TAA), 23
augmentation of, 26-27
Tumor physiology relevance to successful radioimmunodetection, 14-16
Tumor radioimmunodetection, future directions in, 211-232
current problems and potential solutions, 212
strategies for improvement, 213-227
advances in immunoscintigraphic technology and equipment, 225-227
methods for radiolabeling antibodies for immunoscintigraphy, 219-222
selection of radionuclides for immunoscintigraphy, 217-219
targeting agents: antibodies and antibody-like molecules, 213-217
tumor and host characteristics: implications for RID, 222-225

Ultrasound in presurgical staging of colorectal cancer, 92-93